the *Love Body*
SELF-CARE METHOD

More acclaim for
The Love Body:

"This gem of a book is full of practical instructions for building self-compassion and, in turn, a lifestyle that thanks your body and teaches you to 'undiet.' With a focus on mindfulness and loving one's whole self unconditionally, it will show you that you deserve health and happiness."

—Angela Pohl, DO

"Tara provides an assessable approach to improving body wellness—both physically and mentally. A must-read for anyone who wants to engage in a positive relationship with themselves."

—Christine Nefcy, MD

"[A] gentle and straightforward approach to rewire how we think about our bodies, understand the reasoning behind our self-destructive behaviors, and learn to treat ourselves with the grace and compassion that we deserve.

—Andrea Stoecker, DO

the *Love Body*
SELF-CARE METHOD

How to Love Yourself,
Treat Yourself Well, & Be Well!

Tara Rybicki, MS, RDN

MISSION POINT PRESS

Mission Point Press
2554 Chandler Road
Traverse City, Michigan 49696
Tel.: 231-421-9513
E-mail: doug@missionpointpress.com
www.MissionPointPress.com

Printed in the United States of America.

Edited by Brooke L. Diaz

ISBN: 978-1-954786-76-9

Library of Congress Control Number: 2022902654

To my little girls.
I hope I have traveled this path so you never have to.

CONTENTS

My Story: Why I Wrote this Guide   *ix*
Introduction: What is Love Body?   *xiv*

Section 1: Getting Started:
Creating Your Wellness Plan   **1**
- Building self-awareness: Understanding why you do the things you do.
- Section Topics:
  » *Self-reflection: Unwrite your story*
  » *Question your thoughts*
  » *Becoming aware*
  » *Planning for well-being*

Section 2: Nourish, Move, Connect   **17**
- The three Love Body practice pillars: Nourish, move and connect, and the Love Body method techniques including

structured self-awareness activities, knowledge-based information, and planned actions to build into your daily routines.
- Section Topics:
  - » *Self-compassion*
  - » *Mindful living*
  - » *Embodied eating*
  - » *Undieting*
  - » *Eating for mental and physical well-being*
  - » *Exploring movement*

Section 3: Planning for Sustainability   81
- Sustaining body and mind nourishment, self-loving behaviors, and your self-care plan.
- Section Topics:
  - » *Checking in*
  - » *Staying on the path of nourishment*

Appendix   87
- Sample Grocery Shopping Planner
- Balanced Eats and Eating Awareness Journaling Example
- Recipes
  - » *Meal/Sides Recipes*
  - » *Snack Recipes*

Acknowledgments   *115*

About the Author   *116*

MY STORY: WHY I WROTE THIS GUIDE

To tell of the journey that led me to caring for and about myself, I must first tell of my long struggle with body hatred. I recall, more distinctly than I care to, being a young girl, at a neighborhood friend's house, in front of a mirror. As we stood there brushing our hair, I internally cross-examined our faces. Her forehead was shorter and lacked the chickenpox scars of mine, her nose was smaller, her ears were also smaller, her skin was darker, not pale like mine, her hair was thicker; sadly and painfully, in my mind, the list went on. When I got back home, I broke down in tears. The pain was so intense that I can again feel it now. What I wouldn't give to be able to tell that girl that her value is internal and unaltered by external appearance.

And then there was me at the age of 16 in a bathing suit. I remember the level of disgust I had for myself because of the dimpled skin that covered my thighs. My heart ached because I lacked what I perceived as perfection. In my mind, because I lacked this so-called perfection, I was worthless. I felt if my external appearance remained as it was, I could never truly be happy. If only I could sit with that girl now and express that happiness comes from within and is already there waiting to be uncovered. These are just two of countless similar experiences that remain forever etched in my memory.

At the age of 19 I sought help from a therapist. I recall explaining my perception of my body to him — it consisted only of a series of "flaws". He diagnosed me with body dysmorphic disorder. I didn't continue treatment as I was convinced there was nothing wrong with my mind, the problem was solely my body. I never told a single soul that I had received this diagnosis and I desperately tried to bury it from myself as well.

After high school, I studied nutrition in college. Until this course of study I never connected what I ate to how I felt physically and mentally. The concept was completely foreign. The knowledge gained through my coursework caused me to take some serious action to improve my eating. There was so much room for improvement as in college I had been living primarily on pizza dipped in garlic butter, ramen noodles, and beer. Instead, I began eating nourishing foods that made my body feel better and provided a clearer, more positive mindset. I felt stronger, more energetic, I was even motivated to start being physically active, but I still had much more soul searching and learning to do to find true and lasting acceptance for my body.

After college graduation, I began a career as a dietitian. This profession felt so right for me. So many people expressed a desire to lose weight and I now possessed the knowledge to help them do so and in effect create a body they could love. Reflecting back, I can guess that subconsciously I went into this line of work as part of my search for something that would help me love my own body.

Receiving my bachelor's degree did make me feel good about myself and it gave me an idea. If I can't increase my value through this concept of a perfect body, perhaps I can through more achievements. I created distractions from dealing with the core of my self-worth issues by running from achievement to achievement. In retrospect, I know I was using these accomplishments to form some sort of invisible tally of which I was basing my value. The tally never felt high enough or good enough and because of this after completion of one I would nearly immediately start searching for something else I could tackle to improve my perceived value.

Until, that is, Love Body found me. I felt compelled, through what I now realize to be a kismet occurrence, to take on a pet project that involved helping other women create bodies they could love. I teamed up with a partner skilled in life coaching to offer a workshop. As a dietitian, I was to lay the foundation and knowledge of lifestyle habits for our participants to reach their goals. My partner would provide the insights to let these women see their bodies through new, non-judgmental eyes. We called it Love Body.

While I originally thought we were offering the workshop to help only our participants, I found that I too experienced a profound mindset shift. I dwelled on our Love Body tenets regarding personal value being constant, internal, and inherent. The idea that I don't have to base my value off how my body looks, or what others think of me, or what my achievements consist of. That my value just *is*. Through this insight and the many other core concepts of Love Body my eyes opened in a way they never had before.

Through Love Body, something completely unexpected happened within me. What I came to realize was that Love Body was not to teach women how they can create bodies they could love. Not at all, in fact. Rather, it was to create love for the bodies we already have and teach self-caring actions supportive of this love. After decades, through Love Body, I could remove the mask of body disdain I had worn for much of my life. Through Love Body, I no longer tie my previously perceived imperfections to my value or sense of worth. Finally, I am free to treat my body with love and acceptance, as it is, in this moment.

This is my story. I feel it necessary to share the messages of Love Body. I know, professionally, that nutrition and movement are of foundational importance to a healthy body and mindset. I also know, personally, that women like myself need to hear that our bodies don't define who we are and our bodies can be loved as they are. We need to hear repeatedly from childhood on into our adult lives that our bodies are beautiful just the way they are. Our bodies do not need fixing or miracle cures, but rather our bodies are miracles and perform miracles for us each day. The love we can show our bodies does not need to be conditional on outer appearance ... our love for our bodies can and should be strong, consistent, and right now.

INTRODUCTION: WHAT IS LOVE BODY?

*L*ove Body is nurturing yourself, inhabiting your body in a new way, and seeing yourself through fresh eyes. It is learning to tap into a place of self-love that lives within, to take care of yourself fully and accept yourself unapologetically. Love Body *is* that internal place of love. Why take on the work to learn to practice the Love Body Self-Care method? Simply put, to enjoy your body, enjoy your life, and finally… fully be well.

This practice involves principles within three main pillars: Nourish, move, and connect. The topics in these pillars, which are listed below, will teach whole self-nourishment, treating your body well as an act of self-love, self-acceptance and connection with your own inner wisdom.

1. Nourish
   - ♥ Undieting
   - ♥ Embodied eating
   - ♥ Eating for well-being
2. Move
   - ♥ Exploratory movement
   - ♥ Moving for well-being and enjoyment
3. Connect
   - ♥ Mindfulness
   - ♥ Self-Reflection
   - ♥ Self-Compassion
   - ♥ Self-Worth

The Love Body method will guide you through the three pillars above using the following techniques:

- ♥ Structured self-awareness activities
- ♥ Knowledge-based information
- ♥ Planned actions to build into your daily routines

I recommend keeping a dedicated journal to help you with this process, noting your Love Body self-reflections, thoughts, and written activities.

SECTION 1:
GETTING STARTED:
CREATING YOUR
WELLNESS PLAN

Self-observation really is a necessary part of becoming self-aware, which in turn is a prerequisite for sustaining well-being. My own self-observation journey began while at a dietitian conference in Scottsdale Arizona. A fellow dietitian and I decided, after some impromptu Google research, to hike to the summit of Camelback Mountain.

At the beginning, I felt strong and confident. The weather was on our side as it was not too hot or too sunny. We were also well-prepared with snacks, a lot of water, hats, and our hiking shoes. After we got a bit farther in, the terrain became more challenging. The trail hiking turned into more climbing and self-doubt began to take over. My thoughts began telling me, "Well, you definitely can't make it to the summit." On two separate occasions, I stopped and expressed to my climbing partner, "I'm just going to stay here, you go ahead," and "I'll wait, no problem!" She would not allow that. At one point, she felt the same self-doubt while searching for an adequate and safe handhold foothold configuration to get over a high ridge. She turned back and looked at me with only remnants of her previous confidence remaining in her demeanor and said, "I don't think I can do this." I thought to myself, projecting my own self-doubt onto her, "She's right. She can't." Just as I was about to tell her that she was, in fact, correct and we needed to turn around, two other unknown girls screamed from behind us, "YOU GOT THIS!" And that was all it took. She looked at the ridge again, found suitable holds, and propelled herself up and over.

Finally, we reached the summit. I paused and took in the mountaintop and surroundings. To say it was amazing provides a way less than adequate description of that moment. Later I reflected on this experience and it brought so much clarity. My thought that I couldn't make it to the summit was not truth but merely a thought. I did make it. If this thought was not true what other thoughts had my mind told me that were not true? With this self-awareness, I now know the importance of questioning my thoughts as they might not be truth. If I revert to old ways of thinking regarding my body not being good enough, I can question my thoughts and recognize them as false. If my mind tells me that my value is only staked in my physical appearance, I can identify this thought as a lie. And when self-doubt sets in, as it likes to do when challenging situations arise, I can just as well question the thoughts and move past them. I will discuss questioning your thoughts in greater depth later in this section.

SELF-REFLECTION: UNWRITE YOUR STORY

We all have a background that has shaped who we are today. Before you move on to planning for meaningful and sustainable self-care you must take some time to self-reflect. Recognizing what you are currently doing and understanding why you do the things you do is important for moving forward with desirable change. To help you understand your current self, and how you got to where you are, take some time to read your current story about your body. There will be many journaling activities throughout this guide. If you haven't already, be sure to get a journal that you use solely for Love Body activities. Deeply consider and write down your answers to the questions below:

♥ What is your current relationship with your body/food?

♥ What do you do for your body? What does your body do for you?

♥ What are the relationship dynamics?

♥ Is it a fair/healthy relationship?

♥ What is your story about your body? How did you get to this story?

♥ What do you say to your body?

♥ How is your current relationship/story benefitting you?

♥ What need is being met through your current relationship with your body?

With the thought of cultivating change within your mindset here are the Love Body tenets to focus on and record in your journal to keep them in the forefront of your mind:

♥ I have permission to live freely as my beautiful and authentic self.

♥ Happiness is always within me, I can support its manifestation through nourishment, movement, and connection to my inner-wisdom.

♥ My value is constant, inherent, and infinite and not defined by anything externally sourced such as my appearance, comparison to others, or the opinion of others.

♥ I deserve to be well and my body deserves care as it is, in this moment.

♥ Rejuvenation starts with loving and caring action.

Focusing on the above tenets, answer the following questions:

♥ How can you move towards a state of equity in your relationship with your body?

♥ How can you meet your needs in a way that better serves well-being?

♥ How can you look at your body in a loving light?

Because we are drawn to what we are used to, we must use process work as a means of lessening resistance to new habits. What this means is that trying to change the way you think will likely feel uncomfortable and when you are uncomfortable, you may naturally want to stop doing what is making you feel that way. This, however, can lead you to resist the very things that will be supportive of self-care and well-being. But you can learn to engage your resistance mindfully and watch it with a non-judgmental and gentle curiosity. This is the only way to move beyond it. You must be willing to be with the discomfort until the caring thoughts and actions become natural and familiar. Be patient with yourself and the process.

Also, you must recognize that the unhealthy

behaviors that you practice are serving you or protecting you in some way. Investigating and aiming to understand how they are serving you allows you to seek new ways to meet your needs that better serve well-being. Self-reflection is necessary to gain the self-awareness for sustainable self-care. Investigate what it is that you truly need or want. What else can help you meet that need or want that isn't self-defeating? To give one example, perhaps you determine that you crave sweet foods when you are feeling sad. You may choose to find another way to cope with your sadness at the root as you understand the sweet food will not truly help with the core of what is causing the sadness. This is process work and the only thing that will allow it to feel natural is to continue to practice it time and time again.

Here is a self-reflection activity to help you identify patterns that lead to behaviors opposing to self-care:

💜 Practice monitoring your own internal environment. Pay attention to what your internal patterns are that lead to behaviors opposing to self-care:

➤ What physical feelings are you experiencing within your body?

➤ What images are your mind showing you?

➤ Are certain thoughts present?

➤ Are certain emotions present?

➤ Do you notice anything else that leads up to your behaviors?

♥ When you notice these patterns, proactively create a pause prior to the behavior opposing self-care by intentionally moving forward with new actions that meet your needs yet also serve well-being.

♥ With practice this new response will become more natural and automatic.

When you give back to your body through showing it love, it will in turn work even harder for you. When you feel better because of your self-loving actions towards your body, savor and dwell on this improved well-being. Truly stop and take it in at that very moment. Savoring the good can help reinforce continuing the new behaviors.

QUESTION YOUR THOUGHTS

We have a natural tendency to believe the things we tell ourselves. Whether we're defining our value or our ability, we deeply internalize it and hold onto it as truth. For example, if you tell yourself, "I can't be active (or whatever it may be, big or small), it's too hard," then you may not even bother trying. Because of this, it's important to understand your thoughts may not be true and, in fact, may be 100% false. Recall this when thoughts obstruct you from following through with self-caring actions.

Use this self-observation tool with thoughts that are obstructive to your goals:

♥ Acknowledge—Let the thought be present and watch it with curious, non-judgmental observance.

♥ Assess—Question if this thought is truth or not. What other thoughts and feelings co-exist with it? What body sensations? Is there a backstory behind the thought?

♥ Act—If you would like to rewrite it in a way that better serves you, then do so. Move on to take intentional action based on the situation.

In reference to the activity example above, if you can observe this thought and recognize it as false you may choose to rewrite it as, "I will find an activity routine that works for me." You may find making the choice to rewrite this thought makes you better able to set your sights on a routine that does work for you. Accepting self-defeating thoughts as truth without question will prevent you from progressing to where you want to be. Build the following practices into each day to set the foundation for your journey to sustainable self-care. Consider these foundational prerequisites supportive of self-care actions:

Question self-defeating thoughts

Work to center your perspective. When a thought counter-intuitive to what you desire arises, observe and consider converting these thoughts into those that allow for the transformative change you seek as discussed above. Never forget that your value is not defined by your body. The only truth in this respect is that you are more than enough as you are.

Use encouraging self-statements

Make encouraging self-statements strong, true, impactful to your well-being, and relevant to your situation. For example, if you hold the negative concept that you are worthless because you weigh more than you would like to, you may want to create the self-statement, "My value is internal and constant and not in any way connected to my weight." Since this will have to be relevant to your situation and story, it will be different for each person. Once you have your self-statement ready, write it down, keep it visible, and state it aloud each day as frequently as you find helpful. Take some time now to journal your encouraging self-statement.

Visualize yourself following through

Close your eyes and envision yourself taking the necessary steps. Make your visualization detailed and intricate as this can help you identify the necessary steps.

Take intentional action to make it happen

Apart from mindset, following through on planned actions is necessary to cultivate self-care. You will develop a Wellness Plan for intentional action later in this guide.

Know and accept that you will not be perfect

When you feel the need to be perfect, the second you are not you may feel like giving up. This is called all-or-nothing thinking. It's okay to not be perfect and, the truth is, perfection is an illusion. The second you stop trying to be perfect you can allow yourself to breathe when life doesn't go exactly as planned. Some days will be better than others and some days you will not eat as well or move as much as you had hoped. That is okay. Be sure to acknowledge this, in a non-judgmental way, without comparison to others, and then move on.

Realize that changing your body will never bring happiness

True happiness is within you now and can be cultivated through:

- ♥ Showing your body love (eating nourishing food, moving in enjoyable ways, practicing daily self-care).
- ♥ Taking time each day to mindfully savor, in the moment, something amazing that your body is doing for you.
- ♥ Expressing gratitude for the miracles your body performs for you each and every day.
- ♥ Speaking kindly to your body and about it.
- ♥ Avoiding comparison of your body to the

bodies of others. (Comparison of your body to the body of others will rob you of contentment. Your body and your goal are 100% distinct and unrelated to anyone else.)

BECOMING AWARE

Learning to live mindfully takes continuous practice. How I define mindfulness in this guide is an intentional, non-judgmental awareness of what is happening within you and around you in this moment. Focused observance of what is happening in the present moment helps prevent getting lost in painful memories or projecting a future that brings about anxiety, which does not yet and may never exist. Past thoughts or future projections are best used primarily for practical purposes, such as self-observing, visualization, goal-setting, and time management.

Mindfulness can be used to bring your attention to any object of your choosing, whether internal, such as your breath or feelings, or external, such as the flame of a candle or the sound of waves hitting the shore. Using mindfulness to observe feelings specifically can be helpful on many levels. For example, simply actively acknowledging that a feeling is present and observing it non-judgmentally can help you avoid over-identifying with the feeling and ultimately lessen the power that the difficult feeling has over you. It may sound counter-intuitive to draw attention to an emotion that is difficult, but it is in fact the only way to lessen the power of the difficult emotion. The more you run from a feeling the faster it will follow and the stronger it will become.

Mindfulness can be practiced throughout the day in any setting. Here is an activity to begin to get familiar with daily mindfulness involving awareness of pleasant moments. Since happiness can be fostered through gratitude this is a great activity to cultivate not only presence but also joy:

> ♥ Sometime during your day, or several times throughout the day, pause and notice what is pleasant in your environment or in your body. Perhaps there is a gentle breeze, a pleasant sound, a peaceful feeling within, or anything that you would like to focus awareness on. At the end of the day reflect on the pleasant moments as well as the general experience of mindfulness, journal your experiences each day for at least a week. If you enjoy this activity continue to journal it daily.

PLANNING FOR WELL-BEING

Self-care involves nourishing your body and moving your body, beyond this though, a key message to hold close is that of love and acceptance of your body now and always. This love need not be reserved for after you meet a goal you've set but rather should be a constant and infinite love.

In this guide I focus on well-being rather than weight loss. This is because if you are eating mostly nourishing foods, moving your body daily, and applying the other self-loving mindset and mindfulness skills discussed throughout this guide, you are supporting yourself in being healthy, feeling your best, and thriving in this life. Weight and health are independent factors. What makes one thinner doesn't always make them healthier and, likewise, what makes one healthier does not necessarily make them thinner. Healthy bodies come in a diversity or shapes and sizes. Consistent practice of the loving actions noted throughout this guide are more telling of wellness than weight loss. Know this and recall it as often as needed.

For anything to thrive it must be fed. Negativity and hate grow when fed. Love and acceptance can only prevail when nourished. Meaning: Focusing your energy on body hatred will only further perpetuate body-hating behaviors. Rather, focusing on body love helps perpetuate body-loving behaviors. For this reason, acceptance of your current body while you work towards your self-care goals is necessary. Loving your body now will enable you to live your life now, in the present moment. To help evoke this love, recall all the work your body does for you to support and carry you through each day. Also recall that your value is internal and constant and in no way defined by your appearance. Feeding your core being with love will cultivate internal peace. Focus on daily behavioral and environmental changes you can make in the moment that will move you towards greater well-being. Below you will find questions to answer and in doing so you will build your plan to help guide you to loving and caring for yourself. Spend some time reflecting on these questions and journaling your responses to build your plan.

Wellness Plan Creation:

- ♥ What is your vision of wellness? (What would your world look like if you practiced self-caring actions?)
- ♥ What are your current barriers to your wellness vision? (What is currently preventing you from practicing self-care? What are your triggers or internal patterns that lead to behaviors opposing self-care?)
- ♥ What intention would you like to set? (Record a daily intention to help you stay present with this plan. For example: "May I nourish my body, move my body, and show my body love each day.")
- ♥ What behaviors/thoughts/habits will you change to help practice your intention? (Note: Dig deep and assess what need these behaviors are currently serving. Plan to meet this need in a way that better honors self-care and better serves you.)
- ♥ What changes will you make to your

environment to help practice your intention?

💜 What will help you make these changes? (Reflect on a typical day from wake to sleep and note what will help you.)

💜 What positive changes to your physical, mental, or spiritual well-being will occur if you practice your intention?

💜 Now set a reminder to reflect weekly. Know that making adjustments/refinements in your plan as you continue to become self-aware is not only fine but necessary. Keep this plan visible daily as a reminder. How will you recommit to your plan daily?

💜 How/where will you get support when you need it?

Keep this wellness plan visible every day. Keep it alongside your encouraging self-statement in a place that you will see it each day. Continuing to self-observe and build self-awareness is a pivotal part of sustainable self-care.

Complete a check in to reflect on section 1 and journal concepts or activities that you want to recall:

💜 Awareness: Journal your self-reflective notes. What did you learn about yourself?

💜 Knowledge: What information did you gain?

💜 Action: What actions will you move forward with?

15

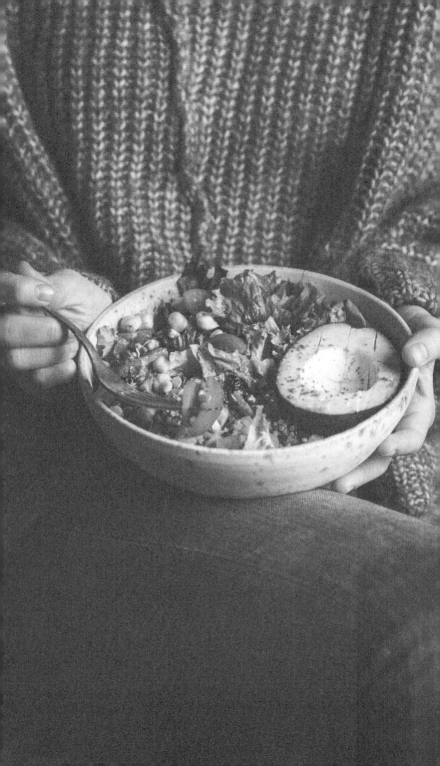

SECTION 2: NOURISH, MOVE, CONNECT

*G*rowing up in a home in the woods, I can easily recall summer days filled with foraging berries, riding bikes and building forts. Eating only when hungry and being active came naturally. At some point a paradigm shift occurred that made listening to my body, eating healthy, and moving my body the anti-norm. I ate very little fruits or vegetables as a teenager and participated in little to no physical activity. Likewise, eating only when hungry and stopping simply because I was full became a foreign concept. I was completely disconnected from my own body. My body was working so hard for me, yet I was doing nearly nothing to show my appreciation and gratitude for its work.

In college, there was ample dorm cafeteria food available and in every variety imaginable. I started off freshman year filling my tray full of everything that sounded even slightly good. It wasn't uncommon for me to eat pizza, ice cream, a sandwich, French fries, chocolate milk, and beyond for lunch and feel sick after doing so. If it was on my tray I finished it, with complete disregard for what my body was telling me. In my dorm I kept a full stock of ramen noodles to eat when the dorm cafeteria wasn't open. And then there was the beer—oh the beer—and then the late-night pizzas to eat after the beer. The college life hit me hard and resulted in a fast and fierce weight gain. So fast in fact that the stretch marks remain on my butt to this day as evidence. During this eating expedition I participated in no activity other than walking to class, which became increasingly harder the longer I mistreated myself. My body sluggishly tried to persevere in supporting me with no reciprocal support from me, and to the contrary, a boatload of abuse.

It wasn't until I gained knowledge through my studies of nutrition that I started giving back to my body and forming a more equitable relationship with it. Understanding the food-body connection was fascinating to me and created the foundation I needed to begin caring for myself and supporting my body. Eating nourishing food gave me a newfound energy and motivation. I begin moving and participating in forms of physical activities that I enjoyed which in turn enhanced my energy even further. Finally, I was providing my body what it needed, and it rewarded me by working even harder to benefit me. It became a beautiful symbiotic relationship.

In this section I will provide this knowledge base by discussing the food-body connection as it relates to getting in touch with the body's cues for hunger and fullness as well as choosing foods that foster physical and mental well-being. This knowledge will fall under the Nourish Love Body pillar. I will also discuss the two other Love Body pillars in the section Move, relating to moving your body as an act of self-love and Connect, relating to connecting to our own inner wisdom, self-acceptance, and self-compassion. We will continue awareness-building activities and planned actions to build this knowledge into your daily life.

SELF-COMPASSION
What is self-compassion?
To me self-compassion is intentionally finding thoughts and actions that reflect kindness, care and acceptance for ourselves. Self-compassion is not selfish, nor is it about letting yourself off the hook because

when you are kind to yourself and care about yourself; you don't give up on yourself. Your food choices are an act of love for yourself. Choosing foods that nourish you is a loving gesture. For the body and mind to support you they need your support. Eating well is a huge part of being well. Likewise, exercise is a part of being well and does not have to be looked at as punishment. Finding movement options that bring you joy and well-being is a loving action that encourages sustainability. Beyond kindness and care, self-compassion is about acceptance. To move forward with any lasting change that involves better serving your well-being you must begin with working on accepting yourself as you are in this very moment. This takes daily reminders, reflection, and so much practice as often self-criticism is the automatic response. Chronic and repeated self-criticism squashes your chance of lasting, sustainable change. It depletes mental resources and shuts down the ability to learn new knowledge and behaviors. With positivity in the brain, you remain open-minded and have access to the area of the mind that allows for logical thought processes and reasoning. To remain free to learn you must foster positivity of the mind.

Self-compassion practice

Mindfulness, self-reflection, and questioning thoughts can help you break free from chronic self-criticism. Try the following activity to bring awareness to any self-critical thoughts, rewire your way of thinking, and halt negative thoughts from being automatic. In turn you will develop a more self-compassionate mindset.

❤ Each day, choose an experience or thought in which you notice yourself being critical, harsh, or negative to yourself and write down the thought. Remind yourself that you do not have to believe the negative thought about yourself. Then, write down something kind you would say to a friend struggling with that same thing and say those kind words to yourself. With time this practice will help self-compassion become more natural and effortless and more automatic over the self-critical path.

LOVE BODY TENETS—ROOTED IN SELF-COMPASSION

The inclusion of these tenets more than once throughout this guide is intentional. We all need consistent reminders of these truths as they build a new mindset as to how we walk through life and how we look at and treat ourselves.

❤ I have permission to live freely as my beautiful and authentic self.

❤ Happiness is always within me, I can support its manifestation through nourishment, movement, and connection to my inner wisdom.

♥ My value is constant, inherent, and infinite and not defined by anything externally sourced such as my appearance, comparison to others, or the opinion of others.

♥ I deserve to be well and my body deserves care as it is, in this moment.

♥ Rejuvenation starts with loving and caring action.

MINDFUL LIVING
What is mindful living?

As mentioned earlier, mindfulness is an intentional, non-judgmental awareness of what is happening within you and around you in this moment. Mindful living is allowing yourself to simply be where you are with kindness and compassion. Being present in this moment gives you freedom from regret or sadness over the past and freedom from anxiety induced from ruminating over the future. Practicing mindfulness each day can help you naturally begin to slow down and provide opportunities to make intentional choices about how you react rather than unintentionally being led around by pre-determined habits. Mindful living can help create new neural pathways and widen the gap between stimulus and response, allowing the ability to choose how to respond from a place of rationality.

Meditation is different than mindfulness in that it is a time set aside to focus awareness on an object such as the breath. A daily meditation practice can help mindfulness become more natural and effortless and integrated in daily life. One way to get started with meditation is to set aside five minutes each day to sit and turn your focus inward. Set an alarm for five minutes, sit comfortably on a pillow or in a chair, and bring your awareness to the sensation of your breath within your body. Each time your mind begins to wander, return your focus back to your breath. Rather than thinking about your breath, focus on the feeling of your breath within your body. When you notice you have become distracted, which is natural, simply redirect your attention back to your breath. This is a great way to train your mind to be present in the current moment and carve out a less reactive pathway, ultimately creating space to choose how you would like to respond to situations before reacting based on urge or emotion. Try this basic meditation practice today.

Speaking personally, this basic daily breath awareness meditations has had profound impact on my stress level and provided me with access to a new, calmer, less reactive pathway to take when encountering difficult emotions or situations. Beyond the aforementioned, depending on the form, meditation may help with several other things such as focus, compassion, mood, outlook, self-awareness, and stress-management.

Grounding techniques help you remain in the present moment and can be especially helpful when things like overthinking or strong emotions are overwhelming you. Growing up my father would often tell me, "Worry is unproductive thought … let it go." This is true and great advice but at that time I unfortunately didn't know how to "let it go." I now know that grounding is the way to release the worry and rumination. Grounding uses your senses to bring you out of our head and back into a calmer state within your body. There are many, many grounding techniques. In this guide I will offer one to get you started. A body scan can be a helpful method for bringing you back to the present moment and into a calmer, more relaxed state. Try this method of grounding:

♥ Love Body scan—practice mindfulness and grounding into the present moment by scanning your body. To do this start by sitting or lying down and then take a deep breath and drop your attention down to your feet. Focus on your feet and any sensations you feel within them. Then focus on bringing loving energy to that area of the body. Feel a warm glow in your feet as the loving energy becomes stronger. Release thoughts or judgements about that area if they do arise. Slowly scan upward from your feet all the way to the top of your head. Stop on each area of the body to feel sensations, bring loving energy to that area, and release thoughts or judgements. For each area of the body try simply noticing without judging. If you choose, this can couple as a self-compassion activity by bringing gratitude and compassion to each area of the body as you scan.

EMBODIED EATING
What is embodied eating?
Embodied eating is intentional, non-judgmental awareness regarding your eating habits, your present moment eating and your food selection. It involves listening to and understanding your body's cues for when to eat and stop eating. It also involves understanding different types of hunger, which I'll explain in depth in this section, and slowing down to make intentional decisions about when to honor hunger. This includes listening and learning what different types of hunger feel like within your body as well as what fullness feels like to you and how to stop eating when full.

Embodied eating involves eating food slowly and thoughtfully and savoring each bite which can bring a new sense of satisfaction and enjoyment to your meals. It also involves taking time to use all your senses to experience the food. This slowing down is of physiologic importance as well. Eating rapidly gives little time for your taste buds to taste and, as such, may not trigger your body's defense mechanism against eating beyond the point of fullness. Also, since it takes your brain, on average, 20 minutes to recognize that your stomach is full, if you eat too rapidly you are set up to eat past the point of fullness.

Embodied eating can bring a completely new awareness and insight to the profound nurturing ability of food as well as allow you to trust in your body's inherent wisdom for what and how much to eat. This in-depth awareness requires the process of daily self-reflection to gain understanding of our current actions. You will find a Embodied Eating Journaling template in the Appendix to help you self-reflect on this daily. Because many of us have tried numerous diets which primarily focus on external cues, such as a calorie level, to drive what and how much to eat, you may be heavily disconnected with your internal cues and at first have a difficult time tuning into them. At first this process can be difficult but know that without intentional choice to take new pathways your pre-determined habits will lead you around and keep you continuing to do things as you always have. Over time and with practice, learning to listen to your body and taking these new pathways will come more naturally. Be patient with yourself and the process as anything new takes time to learn. With daily practice, embodied eating can improve food selection, lessen the likelihood of overeating, and enhance satisfaction in eating. Below is a breakdown of the two broad components of embodied eating: awareness and acceptance.

Embodied eating awareness

♥ Present moment awareness while eating—
   Being present within your body and in

tune with your current emotional state throughout your entire eating experience. Your senses, sight, touch, smell, hearing, and taste can help with embodiment during eating. You can also use intentional focus to check in with your hunger/fullness, situation, and emotional states before, during, and after eating.

♥ Extended awareness related to eating/body—This involves continuous self-reflection to build non-judgmental self-awareness; gauging and understanding what different types of hunger feel like within your body and making intentional, informed decisions about what to eat, when to eat, and how much to eat.

Embodied eating acceptance

♥ Listening to your body, understanding that you need to eat nourishing food to be well, and honoring the need to nourish your body.

♥ Observing your body and food choices from a place of non-judgment, void of self-criticism.

Embodied eating assessment

Answer the following questions to reflect on your level of embodiment in eating:

♥ Do you often eat to soothe or block out emotions/feelings?

♥ Do you often eat when bored or lonely?

♥ Do you have a hard time stopping eating when full?

♥ Do you have a hard time recognizing fullness or hunger or both within your body?

♥ Are you mostly driven by external cues (for example calorie level, presence of food, what others are eating, what diets tell you) for what to eat, when to eat, and how much to eat?

If you *answered Yes* to any of these questions the practice of embodied eating as discussed in this section, including the concepts of pattern interruption, gauging hunger and eating rituals, as well as the Eating Awareness Activity can help get you back to a place of communicating with and listening to your body to guide your eating experiences.

If you *answered No* to all the questions above, then you likely have a high level of embodiment with eating. Continue with embodied eating and other practices that help you maintain this connection to your body.

Self-observation builds awareness in eating

Learning to monitor your internal environment takes a lot of practice. Reflecting can help you identify how your current patterns are serving you and how to carve out new paths that lead to greater well-being.

- 💙 Practice acknowledging and investigating internal cues for hunger and fullness and making intentional decisions about what, when, and how much to eat.

- 💙 Pay attention to certain internal patterns that lead to behaviors opposing self-care. With time, when you notice these patterns within you can proactively create pause prior to the behavior. This pause is important as it allows time to make a choice as to how you would like to proceed as opposed to being led around by pre-determined habits.

You can learn to engage your patterns mindfully and become the watcher of them. Becoming the watcher can be thought of similarly to people watching but the person is yourself and you're watching from within. This is the only way to move beyond habits that aren't serving your well-being. You must be willing to be with things as they are and seek to understand them before you can move on with lasting change. We don't tend to do things unless they meet some need for us. Learning to understand your needs at a core level and meet needs in ways that also serve your well-being takes a willingness to learn about yourself. You can only make changes after you seek to understand your current behaviors through self-reflection. Try the activity below to build a better understanding of your current habits that don't align with self-care or self-love and begin to move beyond them.

Use this journaling activity to explore how your current behaviors are serving you:

- ♥ Self-reflect through journaling to explore what current behaviors you have that don't serve your well-being.
- ♥ Investigate what it is that you truly need at the deepest level. What core need are you trying to meet through your current behaviors?
- ♥ Acknowledge and meet any new understanding that you gain with kindness and supportive thoughts.
- ♥ Explore what else can help meet your needs but also serve well-being.

BEING IN TUNE WITH TYPES OF HUNGER

Emotional hunger

Let's take some time now to discuss emotional eating. This refers to eating food to help cope with or because of an emotion or feeling such as sadness, stress, boredom, or even happiness. Food and water are, of course, critical to life and vitality. As we travel throughout life, we may build emotional connections to food and learn to use food for emotional support. This is very common and some emotional eating may have a place when we make a point to do it mindfully and intentionally. Beyond remaining mindful and self-aware when eating, be sure to have multiple coping mechanisms available that help serve you as you cope with an emotion. If you are aware that you eat emotionally, sit and journal a list of alternate coping techniques that help with emotions. For example, you may find yoga, meditation, going for a walk or talking to a friend to be helpful techniques for coping with stress. Having a multitude of strategies available and on hand helps ensure that you have choices. Whatever the coping technique you use, be sure to let the raw emotions come through and acknowledge them rather than ignoring or subduing them. In the long run, attempting to block difficult feelings and emotions only gives them strength and power over you. Because of this, make a choice to care for these difficult feelings. Also, self-observe to be sure that your frequency of emotional eating is best serving you as opposed to hindering you from being well. Use the embodied eating activity and journaling template in this guide to help you become more self-aware regarding emotional eating. Practice the self-observance discussed and seek the path that helps you with your overall plans for self-care.

To stay in tune with the emotions that are present within you each day, you may find it helpful to add a daily mindfulness check-in of emotions. It could be as simple as setting an alarm that triggers you to stop, take a slow breath in and out, state how you are feeling, and then offer a caring statement for the feeling. For example, if stress is present then you may state, "I acknowledge that I am feeling stress within me." Breathe in and out and state "I am here, in the now." You may find that this brings you back to the current moment rather than caught up in a painful situation from the past or a projection of a future that brings you stress. This is a basic method to try out to help check in on emotions and remind you to seek a coping activity from your list to address the emotion when needed.

Physical hunger

Physical hunger is the physiological response and feeling within the body to hunger. This involves feelings within your body that happen when your body needs food. This may include, for example, stomach growling in early physical hunger and manifestations such as lightheadedness or irritability in later stages of physical hunger. I go in depth on learning to gauge physical hunger and fullness and differentiate physical hunger from other forms of hunger later in this section.

Situational hunger

Situational hunger is often spawned through conditioning. For example, let's say each evening you eat ice cream, you may then be inclined to think about and crave ice cream in the evening whether or not you are truly physically hungry. Another example is if you often eat something sweet after dinner, you may seek something sweet after dinner simply because you are conditioned to want it. One example of situational hunger that I've noticed within myself is that when I am tired, I crave high sugar foods. I also know, through reflection, that it's the energy boost I'm looking for, not really the high sugar food. Because of this, I often choose not to honor this situational hunger and rather find another way to provide energy, whether it be a quick walk or maybe even a nap. Situational hunger may also arise when you see certain foods that you like or even if you smell food cooking. Because this conditioning can easily be set into place it is important to be aware of it so you can make intentional, informed decisions as to whether or not you want to honor your situational hunger. It is also important to have an understanding that using food as a reward system can build situational hunger. For example, if each time you accomplish something you tell yourself you deserve non-nourishing food, you may crave this type of food each time you fulfill an accomplishment. There is nothing wrong with occasionally eating ice cream or pizza or whatever it may be, but when you tell yourself that you deserve these foods because you succeeded at something it can be internally confusing. Whether this confusion is conscious or subconscious it isn't helpful to the overall goal of being well or to the practice of self-care. What you truly deserve is to be well. Rather than rewarding with food, I suggest rewarding with kind and loving words.

Taste hunger

Taste hunger is wanting to eat more of a food because it tastes good to you. Taste hunger can push through physical fullness and make you want to continue eating even when feeling the physiological presence of fullness in our stomach. At times you may choose to honor your taste hunger and eat beyond the point of fullness. Make sure to do this with intentional choice and self-awareness. If you feel that you are being led to eat beyond the point of physical fullness too often due to taste hunger, you may find the embodied eating activity I offer in this section will help you lessen the frequency.

Practical hunger

Now let's move on to discuss practical hunger. There may be times that you may need to eat when you are not necessarily physically hungry. This is referred to as honoring your practical hunger. For example, if you are not necessarily hungry for a 7:00 PM snack but your self-reflection has made you aware that you consistently wake up in the middle of the night starving when you don't eat one, then it is best to eat the 7:00 PM snack. This is simply planning for practical purposes, getting in tune with your body's needs, and setting yourself up to avoid overeating. Or, you may not feel hungry in the morning, but you have self-observed that if you do not eat breakfast you tend to make poor food choices or overeat later; if this is the case then it is best to eat breakfast. This is a part of observing and honoring what works best for your body.

LACK OF AWARENESS IN EATING

In my experience as a dietitian, I've found that what to eat is so frequently talked about on so many platforms. However, how to eat is equally important yet is rarely discussed. The process of building self-awareness and being intentional about our choice of what to eat, when to eat, and how much to eat is necessary for sustainable self-care. As to help further provide understanding of awareness in eating I provide some points on what a lack of awareness in eating may include:

Being disconnected from the body; not checking in with the body

- ♥ Eating at set times regardless of presence of hunger.
- ♥ Not dropping down into your body to feel the stomach and assess hunger.
- ♥ Letting taste hunger take over because you are in a certain situation or because there is food nearby (whether on your plate or in the room).
- ♥ Finishing your food and realizing you barely tasted or even remember eating.

♥ Being guided by strict rules that center around food and eating.

Being engaged in alternate activities while eating
♥ Eating while on electronics.
♥ Standing and/or multitasking while eating.

Emotionally driven eating
♥ Eating to avoid feelings or emotions.
♥ Experiencing guilt after eating certain foods and defining yourself as "good" or "bad" after eating certain foods. Being in a chronic state of negativity hinders change.

PATTERN INTERRUPTION—ADDRESSING WHEN HABITS AREN'T SERVING WELL-BEING

If in reading this section you've identified that eating for reasons outside of physical hunger is a habit that is hindering your well-being, here is an awareness activity to help you identify when you are taking that pathway of your habit prior to following through with it:

♥ *Notice*—identify the circumstances that lead to the habit.
♥ *Ground*—Bring yourself into the present and into your body. When these circumstances arise create pause and draw your awareness to what is happening within your body.
♥ *Soothe*—Find a mantra, imagery, something

to touch or hold, or a movement that helps soothe you as to bring yourself into a calm and rational state of mind.

- ♥ *Seek*—Self-reflect to understand what unmet needs you have (to do this, we need to be in a calm and rational state of mind as opposed to being emotionally driven).
- ♥ *Care*—Choose to proceed in a way that meets your needs AND serves well-being.

GETTING STARTED WITH EMBODIED EATING

Now you are ready to get started with embodied eating. First, begin with a self-reflective journaling activity and record the following:

- ♥ What is your current relationship with embodied eating?
- ♥ What barriers do you have to embodied eating?
- ♥ What are your strengths in relation to embodied eating?

After you have identified barriers and strengths, help set yourself up to make embodied eating more natural by creating a food environment that counters habitual eating. To do this assess the areas that you spend your time and adjust the environment to better serve your well-being. Physically walk through your home and workspace and write down what you would like to change to make embodied eating easier for you.

Also, work to nourish your body throughout the day. Nutrient rich and consistent meals allow you to remain in tune with hunger/fullness. Empower yourself with knowledge on foods that help provide these signals as well. I will provide this information in the *Eating for Well-being* section of this guide. Also, take care of yourself in other ways. This includes getting sufficient sleep and managing stress.

Now to move on with a pre-eating ritual, mid-meal check-ins, and post-eating reflection. This will help ensure that you are making intentional decisions about what, when, and how much to eat as well as getting in tune with your body prior to eating. It involves checking in on hunger level and emotions, breathing to ensure access to rational thought process, chewing thoroughly to help stay in tune with hunger and fullness cues, and a post-eating reflection to determine if there is anything you noticed during this eating experience.

Try this eating ritual at your next eating experience:

Pre-eating:
Begin by sitting down. This sounds like such a small step but the simple act of sitting prior to eating brings a wealth of awareness. Then find a place of authentic gratitude for the food you are about to eat and take a moment to acknowledge that gratitude. After that

take a few deep breaths (fully expelling air) as this will help bring you into a rational state of mind. Lastly, gauge your hunger level, differentiating between physical hunger and other types of hunger discussed earlier.

During eating pause to check in on:

- 💙 Whether you are remaining present within your body rather than distracted or lost in thought.
- 💙 What your level of fullness is in the moment.
- 💙 How you are taking in your food, for example are you eating slowly, savoring and tasting your food, and fully chewing each bite.

Post-eating reflection:

- 💙 What went well during this eating experience?
- 💙 Would you like to change anything during your next eating experience?
  - ➢ What will help you make this change?

LEARNING TO GAUGE YOUR PHYSICAL HUNGER

Even if you have difficulty identifying physical hunger and fullness currently, exploring these body cues can help you get back in tune with them.

Journal your answers to the following questions:

♥ Do you currently feel physical hunger and fullness cues?

♥ What do the different stages of physical hunger and fullness feel like in your body? In your head? In how you respond to life?

To practice getting in tune with your body's physical hunger and fullness signals see the hunger/fullness scale below. This can help in considering what hunger and fullness feel like to you and how to best honor your hunger and fullness.

Hunger scale

Become aware of your body's hunger signals and honor hunger when you are initially to moderately hungry.

♥ No hunger—Neutral state, not hungry or full.

♥ Initial hunger—Food is beginning to sound good; stomach may start gently growling.

♥ Moderate hunger—Thinking about food more, stomach growling.

♥ Extreme hunger—Feeling a sense of urgency with eating, stomach growling and may feel hollow or even hurt, will eat anything available, beyond being comfortably hungry.

➢ Additional physiological symptoms may manifest such as difficulty

concentrating, headache, and low
energy level.

💗 Beyond hunger—Feeling extreme discomfort with hunger level, stomach hurts, may feel panicked in the need to eat.

➤ Additional physiological symptoms may be present such as difficulty concentrating, headache, low energy level fatigue, weakness, dizziness.

Fullness scale

Become aware of your body's fullness signals and stop eating when initially to moderately full.

💗 Initial fullness—Beginning to feel satisfied, may be hungry again in 1-3 hours.

💗 Moderate fullness—Feeling satisfied and comfortable, may be hungry again in 2-4 hours.

💗 Full—Feeling satisfied but would not want to eat more, may be slightly uncomfortable.

💗 Extreme fullness—Feeling discomfort with fullness level, stomach may hurt.

💗 Beyond fullness—Well beyond being comfortably full, may have stomach pains, feeling ill.

At times you may have difficulty stopping eating even when you identify that you are physically full.

Some reasons people eat beyond the point of fullness include:

♥ *Deprivation*—When you deprive yourself of food, you may begin to think about food more often and more intensely. Then, when you do allow yourself to eat, you may have difficulty stopping due to fear of being deprived again.

♥ *Triggers*—These may be environmental triggers such as the presence of food on our plate or perhaps learned triggers such as being taught to ignore fullness and clean your plate, for example.

♥ *Taste hunger*—You may continue to eat beyond fullness when something tastes good to you. This is especially so if it is a food that you tend to deprive yourself of and fear that you won't get to eat it again.

♥ *Lack of awareness*—If you are distracted while eating, you may not recognize that you are full until you are beyond full.

♥ *Rapid eating*—When you eat quickly and do not chew your food thoroughly your mind doesn't recognize that your stomach is full until it is beyond full.

So then, what helps honor fullness and stop eating when initially full? Here are some things that will help:

♥ Including fiber-rich foods and protein-rich

foods in your meals (foods that help identify fullness).

💜 Using a pre-eating/eating ritual.
💜 Learning to gauge what hunger and fullness feel like within your body.
💜 The practice of embodied eating.
💜 Staying present during the experience of eating and checking in with your body throughout.
💜 Slowing down and fully chewing our food.
💜 Giving yourself permission to leave food on plate.
💜 Nourishing your body throughout the day by eating consistently.

Also, eating when you are initially to moderately hungry can help you stop eating when you become initially to moderately full. Waiting until extreme hunger sets in decreases your ability to eat mindfully and increases the likelihood that you will eat to extreme fullness or beyond being full. Also, know that as you begin to practice gauging your hunger and fullness you may notice other signals specific to your body that are not noted in the hunger/fullness scale above. Everyone is different, so use self-observation to become familiar with your body's hunger and fullness cues. The more you practice getting in tune with your body the easier it will be to recognize how your body lets you know it is hungry or full.

CHECKING IN WITH YOUR BODY
ACTIVITY—GAUGING HUNGER LEVEL:

Prior to eating:

- ♥ Close your eyes and get comfortable in your seat.
- ♥ Inhale deeply and exhale slowly. How does your stomach feel? Your head? Your muscles?
- ♥ Take another deep breath and exhale slowly. How do you feel emotionally?
- ♥ Again, inhale and exhale slowly. What are your surroundings?
- ♥ Using the scale above (from beyond hunger to beyond fullness), rate the hunger level of your body. Separate your physical hunger feeling from hunger related to your emotions or environment.
- ♥ What food would you choose right now?

During eating:

- ♥ Use your senses (sight, touch, smell, and taste) to appreciate the food.
    - ➢ Take time to use each sense individually to explore the food.
- ♥ Pause in the middle of eating to re-check the level of your hunger.
- ♥ If your body still feels hungry then eat more. If you are comfortable then stop.

❤ Try to recognize when your body begins to feel full.

   ➤ What are your body's signals that you are comfortable and becoming full?

Incorporate this activity into your daily meals as often as possible. With practice it will become more automatic to recognize hunger and fullness cues and learn to identify physical hunger, emotional hunger, and situational hunger. Practicing this technique can make embodied eating become more natural and effortless. If you feel completely out of tune with what hunger and fullness feel like, refer to the scale of physiological feelings associated with each mentioned earlier. If your hunger and fullness cues are not prevalent, perhaps due to chronic dieting, know that with continued practice of nourishing your body throughout the day they will return. After you become familiar gauging your hunger level with the activity above, transition to the following more comprehensive embodied eating practice:

EMBODIED EATING ACTIVITY:

Prior to plating your meal/snack:

   ❤ Close your eyes.

   ❤ Inhale deeply and exhale slowly. Take stock of your body: How does your stomach feel? Your head? Your muscles?

   ❤ Take another deep breath in and exhale

slowly. Take stock of your feelings: How do you feel emotionally?

♥ Open your eyes. Again, inhale and exhale slowly. Take stock of your environment: What are your surroundings?

♥ Using the scale provided earlier (from beyond hunger to beyond fullness), rate the hunger or fullness level of your body. Distinguish your physical hunger feeling from hunger related to your emotions or environment.

♥ Consider the vast nourishing capacity of food to give you energy, to keep you alive, and help you thrive physically and mentally.

♥ Ask yourself the following: What food will you choose right now? Why are you choosing this? Are you seeking food to fill a need outside of physical hunger? If so, how can you meet that need at the root? How will eating this make you feel?

♥ Portion out the amount of food you think will satisfy you.

♥ Sit down with the food, taking a few deep breaths, focus solely on the moment you are in and on the food you are about to eat. What else may help you eat with awareness?

♥ Take time to reflect appreciation for the

food you are about to eat. Find a place of authentic gratitude and consider all that it took for this food to get to your plate.

During eating:

- ♥ Use your senses (sight, touch, smell, and taste) to appreciate the food. Take time to use each sense independently to explore the food.
- ♥ First touch the food. Consider how it feels between your fingers.
- ♥ Then look at the food. What do you notice about it? Now look even closer and observe it even more deeply.
- ♥ Next hold it close to your nose. Can you observe any smell from it?
- ♥ Now, take a bite of the food. Prior to chewing, roll it around in your mouth a bit and explore the taste as well as any mouth sensations it may bring. Pause and let yourself fully take in the taste and the experience of eating.
- ♥ Continue to eat while focusing your awareness solely on the food. Chew each bite thoroughly and pay attention to the flavor and sensations it brings within the body.
- ♥ Pause in the middle of eating to re-check the level of your hunger. Stay connected

and in tune to your body and what it is telling you.

- ♥ If your body still feels hungry then eat more. Even if it is more than you originally portioned out. If you are comfortable stop. Even if there is still food on your plate.
- ♥ Try to recognize when your body begins to feel comfortable.
  - ➤ What are your body's signals that you are comfortable and becoming full?

After eating:

- ♥ Using the fullness scale provided earlier, rate the fullness level of your body immediately after you finish eating. How do you feel physically? How do you feel emotionally?
- ♥ The intention is to be satisfied without being overly full. Listening to your body can help you stop eating when you are starting to feel full or when you feel satisfied without feeling overly full.
- ♥ Is there anything you will change the next time you eat?
- ♥ What can support you in building embodied eating into your habits and life?

Another suggestion that can be helpful to add to embodiment in eating is to designate specific areas to use solely for eating, for example, the dining room table would organically fit this purpose. When eating at home, use this designated area and focus solely on food without doing other activities. To help with this, make it habit to turn off the television and set aside your phone while eating. Also, you will find an Eating Awareness Journaling example in the Appendix. Using this as a template for daily journaling will help build self-awareness and make embodied eating naturally integrate into your routine.

It is also important that you acknowledge when you are not present within your body during your eating. If you recognize that you are not practicing embodied eating, acknowledge, take a deep breath, and bring yourself back to the moment. It is okay and no one is perfect, nor should you expect yourself to be. If you notice you have already overeaten, actively acknowledge this and move on. Objectively state what the circumstance is without placing judgement on yourself. For example, "I overate and I feel uncomfortable and a bit sick." If you ate the amount that made you feel satisfied without being overly full, then acknowledge that and state how that made you feel. For example, "I practiced embodied eating and feel satisfied and comfortable." Describe the facts objectively rather than placing any judgment. This acknowledgment is a part of self-observance and will help you become more self-aware. Embodied eating is a daily practice rather than a one-time event so be patient with yourself.

At times, you may make an intentional choice to eat when distracted or make an intentional choice to eat beyond the point of physical hunger. You may also make an intentional choice to eat to comfort an emotion. This is your choice. Embodied eating is about finding balance. When you start to establish strict food rules around embodied eating then it may begin to feel like just another unsustainable diet. As such, this may lead to the diet cycle of over-restriction to feelings of deprivation to overconsumption to feelings of guilt and then back to over-restriction. Sadly, this cycle seems infinite and this is why we must consciously decide to not establish strict rules around embodied eating.

UNDIETING
What is undieting?
Undieting is removing your focus from weight or another outcome that involves changing your body. Instead, you place your attention on taking care of your body and practicing self-loving behaviors. Undieting involves building self-awareness, gaining a new knowledge, and intentional action.

Awareness
Self-reflection is necessary to become self-aware. Reflecting can help you identify how your current patterns are serving you and how to carve out new paths that lead to greater well-being. Reading your story is

the only way to rewrite your story, meaning the way to initiate habit change is to become the watcher of yourself. Below are some opportunities for reflection. Take your time to work through each to bring self-awareness related to undieting.

♥ Journal your current barriers and strengths regarding undieting. Explore your environmental barriers and core barriers and beliefs. Environmental barriers refer to those things within your environment that make this process difficult. Core barriers, which may take a lot of time to unveil and reveal to yourself, are those barriers that are deeply embedded within you and your beliefs. For example, maybe your core barrier to undieting is that you were taught that unless you are thin you have no value. Or perhaps, you feel that you don't deserve to be well so you sabotage yourself. Or you may have been deprived of food as a child so feeling even slight hunger may bring up unconscious fear. Or you may even be drawn to pain and suffering so when things are too calm in your environment you subconsciously seek out situations or act in ways that will cause you to suffer. Without addressing the core barriers blocking you from any behavior change you will not be able to move beyond them.

So, spend a lot of time journaling and discovering your own core barriers.

♥ Because as a society we are conditioned to diet, do some journaling and exploration around the following questions:

➤ Are you ready to reject dieting?

➤ How will rejecting diet culture challenge you?

➤ How does dieting serve you?

➤ How might your life improve if you reject diet culture?

♥ Self-compassion is a necessary part of undieting and involves:

➤ Releasing perfectionism—Accepting yourself as you are in the current moment relieves great pressure and can perpetuate self-caring actions.

➤ Caring for yourself—When you truly care about yourself, you want well-being for yourself and thus practice actions that bring you well-being and health.

➤ Absence of self-criticism—Repetitive self-criticism naturally brings fear. This fear halts you from planning efforts that bring health and well-being as you learn to think if you fall short, you are inherently bad. This is false. One common example I hear as a dietitian is, "I ate poorly today so I might as well continue to eat poorly." This all-or-nothing thinking is damaging to your intention for self-care. Each new moment offers new opportunities to care for yourself and be well.

➢ Reflecting on your level of self-compassion.

💜 Releasing the sole focus to an outcome of eating that involves changing the body size or shape and shifting your primary focus to that of nourishment and caring action for your body.

➢ This also involves releasing the "if only I can lose weight, I will be happy" mindset. Rather know that cultivating lasting joy happens through:

💜 Showing your body love through self-loving actions.

💜 Mindfully living in the now.

💜 Expressing gratitude every single day.

💜 Speaking kindly to and about yourself.

💜 Avoiding comparison of yourself to others.

💜 Internalizing the fact that value lies within you and releasing the need for external validation of value.

➢ Explore whether you are an external validation seeker. An external validation seeker gets perceived value from what others think or say. Recall that self-worth is inherent and constant within you. Positive feedback from others does not increase your value just as negative feedback from others does not decrease your value. Cultivating mindset shift to accept the truth that value is unwavering may take a lot of time. Use the Love Body tenets as a daily reminder.

♥ Exploring your current rules around food and releasing those that do not serve well-being. Reflect on the following:

➢ What diet culture influenced rules do you have around food and eating?

➢ How did you get these rules?

➢ What will help you release rules that do not serve your well-being?

Knowledge

In relation to undieting, this involves empowering ourselves with the knowledge of the foods that nourish and keep us in tune with hunger and fullness cues. To help yourself build a knowledge base in this area read the section on eating for well-being. Also, continue with the practice of embodied eating that you learned earlier. Re-learning to listen to your body and allowing your eating to be guided primarily by your internal cues takes time and patience so grant yourself grace.

Action

There are many intentional actions that aid in living a lifestyle free from diet culture. Here are some to help guide you:

- ❤ Eating with the intention of both nourishing and caring for the body and mind.
- ❤ Practicing caring for the body in the present moment and reciprocating the care the body provides you.
- ❤ Taking intentional action towards well-being and planning for sustainability. To help build structure around this use the wellness and sustainability plans in this guide.
- ❤ Understanding this is a practice—meaning it is a lifelong process.
- ❤ Finding comfort in discomfort:
  - ➢ Understanding resistance to change— we are drawn to what we are used to so we may be resistant to change even if the change better serves our well-being. Because of this you must be willing to sit with the discomfort and allow time for the new habits to

become a new norm and begin to feel less foreign and uncomfortable.

➤ Curiosity—Investigate your discomfort and allow it to be present.

➤ Soothe—Find things that help soothe the discomfort. Some examples of soothing gestures include grounding techniques, kind words to yourself, sensations such as placing your hand on your heart or stroking your arm, moving your body, or visualizing calming images. This can help cultivate calm in the uncertainty and foreignness of new habits.

♥ Learning to be at home in the moment and less reactive—allowing discomfort to be present and soothing yourself during these times of discomfort rather than distracting from them or criticizing yourself during them.

THE "WHY NOT" OF FAD DIETS

It is important to distinguish between therapeutic, medically necessary diets and fad diets. Therapeutic diets are needed due to a medical condition. For example, if you have Celiac disease, you must follow a gluten free diet for health and well-being. Therapeutic diets help with treatment of a condition and therefore are necessary. When I discuss undieting I am not referring to undieting from medically necessary diets. I am referring to releasing yourself from fad dieting. Fad diets center around eating recommendations provided with the intention of purporting information to tell others how to lose weight. However, these diets are designed with the wrong intentions: making a profit for those who develop them. They are a completely unsustainable way of eating and because of this they don't work in the long run. Fad diets do offer a temporary fix … typically leading to a rapid weight loss followed by a regain of the weight. Each time you go through the lose-regain cycle, it potentially weakens your metabolic rate. This diet cycle is not your fault as fad diets set us up to feel deprived. Intense cravings and urges to eat are the body's natural response to feelings of deprivation. These cravings and urges will cause you to eat and perhaps even binge on the foods you are craving. This leads to regaining any weight that you may have initially lost. Simply put: Fad diets don't work.

WHY UNDIETING IS A BETTER WAY

Here is a list of undieting words vs fad dieting words that will help you differentiate:

Undieting
- 💜 Trust
- 💜 Permission
- 💜 Empowerment

- ♥ Internal cues
- ♥ Well-being focused
- ♥ Acceptance
- ♥ Flexible
- ♥ Nourishment
- ♥ Balance
- ♥ Lifestyle
- ♥ Sustainable

Fad-dieting

- ♥ Will power
- ♥ Denial
- ♥ Obedience
- ♥ External cues
- ♥ Weight loss-focused
- ♥ Control
- ♥ Rigid
- ♥ Avoidance
- ♥ Restrictive
- ♥ Trend
- ♥ Food fear promoting
- ♥ Unsustainable

But what should I weigh?

As mentioned prior, place your attention on caring for your body and practicing self-caring behaviors. Release strong attachment to future outcomes that involve losing weight or changing your body. Put your focus on the love and care you are providing for yourself while you are nourishing and moving your body each day. When you treat yourself well you can become well without focusing on the number on the scale.

To help you do this recall the section on questioning your thoughts and try this daily mindfulness exercise for breaking down untruths:

♥ Noticing untruths—We all tell ourselves things that are not true at times. We must notice these untruths or they can rule the day, the week, or even years. So, notice when you tell yourself something that is not true about your body and then counter it with a true, compassionate statement. An example of an untruth related to body may be, "I have cellulite and that makes me unworthy of love and care." A compassionate counter statement to this may be, "Cellulite is natural, my body deserves my care and love as it is in this very moment." Spend at least a week journaling the untrue statements that you hold about your body and the compassionate statement that you counter it with.

Examining reference points will also help you release attachment to weight loss. If you follow a lot of workout influencers on social media for example, then you begin to believe this is what you should look like. Likewise, if you often read fitness magazines you may feel as though this is what your body should look like.

If you notice an imbalance in reference points for what bodies look like, you must do the work to create balance. Unfollow the workout influencers and dieting platforms and follow those focused on well-being in body and mind. Stop purchasing workout magazines and, rather, read articles that will aid you on your journey to care for yourself truly and deeply.

EATING FOR MENTAL AND PHYSICAL WELL-BEING

Your food choices are an act of love for yourself. Choosing foods that nourish you is a loving gesture. For the body and the mind to support you they need your support.

Nourish the body and mind

Several supportive nutrients offer protection against pathways that may make us more likely to develop chronic illnesses such as type 2 diabetes, heart disease, and some cancers and mental illnesses such as anxiety and depression. Setting yourself up to be strong, well, and resilient starts with providing nourishing food choices. Shift the inner dialogue from eating nourishing food to change your body or lose weight to eating nourishing food to show yourself love and encourage well-being. Bear in mind that eating, and life in general, is about balance. Finding this balance is a part of building self-supporting behaviors that are sustainable throughout life. It is ultimately your choice to mindfully select the foods you eat. This section is to provide an informational base on nutrition to help you make informed food decisions. On the occasions that you choose foods that are not nourishing do so without negativity towards yourself or your actions. Negative thoughts about yourself only perpetuate behaviors that are not supportive of self-care.

Examples of protective nutrients:

- ♥ Omega 3 fatty acids
- ♥ Antioxidants
- ♥ Probiotics/Prebiotics
- ♥ Vitamins/Minerals
- ♥ Fiber

Potential protective effects related to diet:

- ♥ Anti-inflammation
- ♥ Protection from oxidative stress
- ♥ Supporting a thriving gut microbiome
- ♥ Support of body processes and metabolism

Supportive nutrients

Having a deep understanding of how foods promote physical and mental well-being in the body can provide reason and motivation to eat these foods and help understand the self-caring action of nourishment. Let's discuss some of the nourishing compounds and foods that contain them. Beyond being nourishing, as they contain vitamins, minerals, antioxidants, omega 3s, and probiotics/prebiotics, they also include components such fiber, protein, and healthy fats to help the body recognize fullness. This is important as the sensation of fullness can be hard to get back in tune with after following dieting rules for how much to eat as opposed to listening to the body. The goal of this discussion is solely to provide practical, evidence-based information. Providing your body with nutrients that it needs enables your body to support your well-being. Also, this is not a diet, so foods that are not mentioned need not and should not be cut out. This is neither an all-inclusive or an exclusive list. Whatever foods you choose, do so with awareness and acknowledgement. It is important to learn to eat in balance. Recall that this guide is not about punishment, deprivation, or starvation. To the contrary, it is about nourishing your whole self and caring for yourself. Aim to eat the nourishing foods often, get back in tune with your body signals for fullness and hunger, and practice listening to what your body is telling you. Moving on, as to further your informational base, discussed below are some food components, how they work to nourish your body, and foods that contain them. This is not a comprehensive list of beneficial food compounds and nutrients, rather it is calling out some specific beneficial compounds found in foods.

Omega 3 fatty acids

- ♥ Reduce inflammation in the body, may lower triglyceride levels, may improve symptoms for those with depression and anxiety, and potentially reduce the risk of dementia.

- ♥ Examples of omega-3 fatty acid containing foods:
  - ➢ Chia seeds
  - ➢ Fish, such as salmon
  - ➢ Flaxseed, milled
  - ➢ Walnuts

Antioxidant/Phytonutrients

- ♥ May have a protective or regenerative effect on cells and may lower the risk of certain diseases, such as cancer.
- ♥ Examples of antioxidant containing foods:
  - ➢ Beans
  - ➢ Chia seeds
  - ➢ Dark chocolate / cacao
  - ➢ Flaxseed, milled
  - ➢ Fruits
  - ➢ Lentils
  - ➢ Nuts and seeds
  - ➢ Oats
  - ➢ Tea, such as green tea
  - ➢ Vegetables
  - ➢ Whole grains

Probiotics/Prebiotics

- ♥ Help build healthy bacteria in your gut (thriving microbiome) and, as such, may enhance immunity and defend against illness. A thriving gut microbiome is an important piece of the puzzle to achieving a nourished body. And consuming a variety of these foods consistently can help in modulating the gut microbiome to your benefit, cultivating a more diverse microbiota. A favorable ecosystem in the gut has been associated with immunity, metabolism, and mental health. Also, the gut microbiota plays a critical role in digestion of food, making essential vitamins accessible to the body and protecting the body from illness. Favorable gut microbiota can also prevent compromised integrity of the gut lining. This is important because a compromised gut lining allows food particles and toxins into the bloodstream which in turn can trigger chronic inflammation and certain diseases. Below I will discuss fermented foods, probiotics, and prebiotics, what they are, how they differ, and why are they important.

♥ Examples of probiotic/prebiotic containing foods:

➢ Fermented foods are made by using a controlled method of microbial growth and activity. This process acts to preserve the food and has the potential to promote health when consumed. The fermentation process can produce beneficial food aspects. For example, it may lower anti-nutritional compounds and result in new beneficial products such as B vitamins (folate, riboflavin, B12, depending of the strain of bacteria present), beneficial bacteria, and vitamin K2 which is thought to play a part in disease prevention and is different and distinct from the vitamin K1 found in green leafy vegetables. The bacteria produced by fermentation may also produce compounds that show antioxidant effects and/or prebiotic properties. In some fermented foods, the beneficial bacteria are killed during post fermentation processing. To help ensure that the beneficial bacteria are present, choose fermented foods that include "living" cultures when available. Fermented foods can be incorporated into your eating habits gradually over time to lower the potential for digestive issues. Examples of fermented foods:

- ♥ Kefir
- ♥ Kimchi
- ♥ Kombucha
- ♥ Miso
- ♥ Sauerkraut

♥ Some cheese (aged, soft)
♥ Tempeh
♥ Yogurt

➢ Probiotics are living microbes that have a health benefit when consumed. There are several different genus, species, and strains of probiotic cultures. To give an example, in the probiotic Lactobacillus rhamnosus GG, Lactobacillus is the genus, rhamnosus is the species, and GG is the strain. Research has shown that different genus/species/strains of probiotics may have completely different benefits in our bodies, one being enhanced immunity against illness, which is quite fascinating if you think about it. A healthy gut microbiome may be supportive of overall health, disease prevention, and immunity against illness. Examples of probiotic foods:

♥ Some fermented foods (see above) noted to contain living cultures and have a proven health benefit.

➢ Prebiotics act as food for the beneficial bacteria of your gut, known as probiotics. Having adequate amounts in the diet can help support a healthy and a thriving gut which, as mentioned above, can in turn be supportive of health. Examples of prebiotic foods:

- ♥ Apples
- ♥ Asparagus
- ♥ Bananas
- ♥ Barley
- ♥ Flaxseed
- ♥ Garlic
- ♥ Jerusalem Artichoke
- ♥ Leeks
- ♥ Onions

Fiber

- ♥ Fiber offers amazing benefits such as promoting a healthy body through regular bowel movements, lowering cholesterol, and regulating blood glucose. Also, fiber holds food in the stomach longer by delaying gastric emptying. When food is in the stomach longer it allows foods to naturally let us know when we are satiated making it easier to identify and respect hunger and fullness cues. Above all this, it may be linked to cancer prevention for certain types of cancer.
- ♥ Examples of fiber containing foods:
  - ➢ Beans
  - ➢ Chia seeds
  - ➢ Flaxseed, milled
  - ➢ Fruits

- ➤ Lentils
- ➤ Nuts and seeds
- ➤ Oats
- ➤ Whole grains
- ➤ Vegetables

Vitamins and Minerals

- ♥ Some vitamins help with the utilization of carbohydrates, proteins, and fats in the body.
- ♥ Vitamins and minerals are involved in many body processes. This includes blood pressure and sugar regulation; brain function; digestion; growth/development; heart function; hormones; immune function; metabolism drugs/toxins/food; muscle contraction; nervous system function; red blood cell formation; reproduction; taste/smell; vision; wound healing.
- ♥ Vitamins and minerals also play an important part in prevention of acute and chronic disease.
- ♥ Examples of vitamin and mineral-containing foods:
  - ➤ Beans
  - ➤ Eggs
  - ➤ Fish
  - ➤ Fruits & Vegetables
  - ➤ Lentils

- ➢ Nuts & seeds
- ➢ Poultry
- ➢ Whole grains

Vitamins and Minerals specific to mental well-being

- ❤ When discussing food choices what is often left out is how supportive nourishing foods can be for our mental health. When looking at well-being and resilience it is essential to build a strong foundation, not only physically but also mentally. Because of this I want to point out some specific vitamins and minerals that may help with mental well-being.
- ❤ B vitamins such as B12, B6, and folate.
  - ➢ B12
    - ❤ Eggs
    - ❤ Salmon
    - ❤ Tuna
    - ❤ Nutritional yeast
  - ➢ B6
    - ❤ Chickpeas
    - ❤ Fruits
    - ❤ Potatoes
    - ❤ Salmon
    - ❤ Tuna
  - ➢ Folate
    - ❤ Asparagus
    - ❤ Avocado

- ❤ Leafy greens
- ❤ Legumes
❤ Magnesium
  - ➤ Almonds
  - ➤ Avocados
  - ➤ Bananas
  - ➤ Beans and peas
  - ➤ Cacao
  - ➤ Leafy greens
  - ➤ Seeds
❤ Vitamin D
  - ➤ Egg yolks
  - ➤ Fish
  - ➤ Fish liver oil
  - ➤ Fortified dairy and other products
  - ➤ Some mushrooms
❤ Zinc
  - ➤ Beans and peas
  - ➤ Nuts
  - ➤ Poultry
  - ➤ Seafood
  - ➤ Whole grains

Take a moment to reflect on how these nutrients can help your body thrive. Recall this as you move forward on your path to practicing holistic self-care. When choosing foods, remember to choose nourishing options that support your body and make it work even harder for you.

THE PHYSIOLOGY BEHIND BALANCED EATING

Meal planning and mindfulness can co-exist. Planning for practical purposes can be helpful as it sets us up with the foundation we need to make self-loving behaviors more effortless and integrated into our daily routine.

Getting the proper nourishment provides the fuel your body needs to have energy and thrive. Eating nourishing foods consistently throughout the day helps ensure that you get adequate nutrients and avoid becoming overly hungry. When you become overly hungry it is naturally difficult to eat with awareness. Nourish your body throughout the day to prevent deficiencies, to stabilize hunger level, to maintain energy, and to encourage both mental and physical health. As always, complete your hunger check prior to eating and let embodied eating guide your food intake. Remember to honor both hunger and fullness and to honor your practical hunger when needed.

Including a satiating mix of foods at meals and snacks can help with stabilization of hunger level, making it easier to honor hunger and fullness cues. Including high fiber foods (such as vegetables, fruits, whole grains, and beans) paired with foods that have protein and healthy fats can help the body feel fullness as this holds food in the stomach longer. This slow emptying of food from the stomach also results in more stable blood glucose and insulin levels which helps to prevent dramatic shifts in hunger and energy level. So for physiological reasons, eating these foods helps you connect with your body's hunger and fullness cues. Protein can further get you in tune with fullness cues by decreasing the body's hunger hormone to provide additional physiological signals to stop eating when you are becoming full.

To help include high fiber foods with proteins and healthy fats for the satiating mix discussed above I offer the following table which includes ½ your meal as vegetables & fruits, ¼ meal grains & starches, ¼ meal protein, and inclusion of healthy fat. Note that this is simply a tool, not a rule, that you may find helpful for balancing meals in a way to help the body identify fullness and stabilize hunger. If you think this will be a helpful tool I have included a *Balanced Eats* chart in the appendix that further details this.

Grocery shopping activity

As the next step in your journey it is important to take some time to plan a research trip to the grocery store with the goal of trying new nourishing foods that sound enticing to you, making some new recipes that you think you'll love, and viewing the grocery store through new eyes—noticing different items you haven't looked at in the past. To do this, start by finding some foods and recipes that sound good (you can use the recipes in appendix if you'd like). Next, get your grocery shopping list together (see sample grocery list in appendix) and then head to the grocery store with your list. Grab a coffee or tea and make it a fun, leisurely, and enjoyable trip with plenty of time allotted to get the items you planned as well as look at new items. After you've tried out some new foods and recipes journal your answers to the following:

- ♥ What were the positives of trying new foods?
- ♥ What were the negatives of trying new foods?

You can continue to try new foods by making it a point to add these "research" trips to the grocery store monthly. Give foods a chance and try them in new ways, but if there is a food that you simply do not like know that you do not have to eat it. What you eat is your choice. Beyond this, know that you must give yourself permission to eat all foods. Practice eating in balance. If you are at a wedding and would like some cake, eat the cake. Check in first to ensure that you even do truly want the cake. Food should not be feared. Create a balance that is desirable to you but also supportive of self-care.

To help keep nourishing choices easily accessible to you, here are some suggestions:

- ♥ Have easy go-to recipes on hand that include foods that you love—I have provided several recipes in the appendix for you to pick and choose from.
- ♥ Prepare extra and freeze for later.

- ♥ Invest in kitchen tools that will help prepare healthy meals, for example a crockpot.
- ♥ Choose items that don't require much prep.
- ♥ Include vegetables or fruits with most meals and snacks.
- ♥ Purchase a lunch box and water bottle to assist with pre-planning and packing.
- ♥ Have a grocery list—In the appendix I offer the grocery shopping list I created that works well for my family. I offer this as an example. Feel free to use it or to create your own. When creating a grocery list, I find it helpful to break the list into sections of the grocery store. This ensures you aren't running back and forth across the store several times.
- ♥ Practice flexible meal planning and use your ideas to inform your grocery shopping list:
  - ➤ Meal planning, when used in a flexible way, can be a helpful and practical tool to support structure, make life less stressful, and perhaps even open time to allow for more mindful meals. However, when used rigidly and as another external cue for when and what to eat, it can distract from getting in tune with the body's internal

cues and become just another unsustainable way of eating. Be sure your meal planning allows for adjustment.

Environmental assessment activity

Being surrounded by an environment that is not supportive of your well-being will make it very difficult to continue this path. Some examples of unsupportive surroundings include those that set you up to eat non-nourishing foods often, act in ways that do not support health, limit your ability to be physically active, create internal feelings of chaos, enhance stress, or distract from self-care including getting adequate sleep. Assessing your environment and actively doing what you can to cultivate an environment supportive of well-being will help fully embrace your self-care practice. To do this assessment, slowly go room by room in your home and work settings and write down two lists:

1. What is *helping* you with self-care?

2. What is making it *difficult* to care for yourself? Next, work to change your environment. Write down things you will continue from your "helping" list and think of ways to add to that list. From the "difficult" list, what can you remove? Simply:

- 🖤 Remove
- 🖤 Continue
- 🖤 Add

EXPLORING MOVEMENT
Finding your why—changing your movement mindset

You can move your body with the intention of caring for your body in the moment rather than the intention of changing your body in the future. Moving your body helps the body in so many ways beyond losing weight. Spend time investigating your own personal why behind moving your body. Aside from losing weight, place your focus on how moving benefits your: strength, health, well-being, energy, vitality, happiness. Use this focus to build a why that is meaningful to you—finding your why helps provide reason to treat yourself well and continue moving. Journal your answers to the following questions to build self-awareness:

- 💜 In a typical day, in what kinds of ways do you move your body?
- 💜 What types of movement/physical activity bring you joy?
- 💜 Does a desire to change your body affect your movement choices?
- 💜 As you move through the day, are you aware of your body, are you experiencing your life through your body or are you primarily in your head?
- 💜 Do you ever acknowledge gratitude for your body's capabilities?

♥ What will help you to move your body each day?

Releasing all-or-nothing thinking

All-or-nothing thinking will stop any self-care plan from being sustainable. All-or-nothing thinking is the mindset that if I did not do what I had planned to move towards my goals, then I might as well not do anything. The fact is that there will be times that your day won't go as planned and there will be days where you didn't do any of the things that you had hoped to do for self-care. Build awareness around this and reflect to see if you have fallen victim to this line of thinking.

Because life is unpredictable, you may find it helpful to develop your "If Nothing Else" strategy. This is a daily movement activity that you know you can do regardless of what your day looks like. For example, maybe you aim to dance for 40 minutes each day as a part of your wellness plan but your "If Nothing Else" is that you will dance to one song. Another example may be that you have a goal to jog for 30 minutes, your "If Nothing Else" could be that you will walk for 15 minutes. This can help reduce the feeling of self-defeat that may come with not being able to complete your broader goal. You can also set an "If Nothing Else" in relation to eating and meditation.

Be flexible and gentle with yourself but also remember you deserve to be well and wellness takes caring actions. Ultimately, any movement is a wonderful form of self-care. Find what you love and do that. To find what you love the key is to seek out fitness opportunities you want to try and commit to trying them. Then, once you have found what you like, incorporate it into your wellness plan.

Daily movement exploration

When exploring movement, start small and keep it simple and doable. Investigate different forms of movement that you think you may enjoy. For example, if you think you may enjoy dancing try a dance class, dancing video, or put on music and dance to that. Or maybe you already know what you enjoy but gave up on it because you weren't losing weight. Maybe you enjoy strength training because it makes you feel strong and empowered. Whatever the type of movement, release the attachment to the outcome of weight loss and focus on the care you are providing for your body in the moment that you are moving. Make a list of different types of movement that you want to try out and then try them. Continue to do whatever forms of movement you enjoy and feel good to you. When you find yourself getting discouraged or down on yourself, recall your why. Change the narrative to one in which you move your body to care for your body in this moment rather than change your body in the future. What movement type will you commit to this week?

Complete a check-in to reflect on section 2 and journal concepts or activities that you want to recall:

- ♥ Awareness: Journal your self-reflective notes. What did you learn about yourself?
- ♥ Knowledge: What information did you gain?
- ♥ Action: What actions will you move forward with?

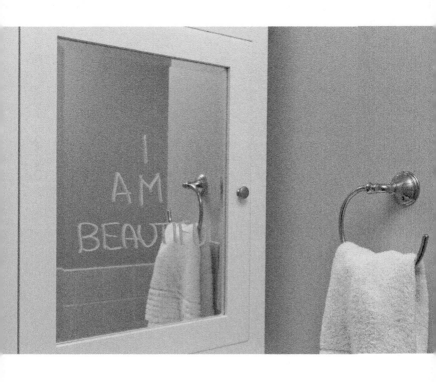

SECTION 3: PLANNING FOR SUSTAINABILITY

I feel significant gratitude that Love Body found me. While I will never be able to go back to the younger me, struggling with a devastatingly poor body image, to teach her these concepts I can speak the tenets and teachings to other women now. I can live this life of body acceptance and model this for my own little girls. I can do my small part in this world to show that there is a different way of thinking about ourselves and our bodies. I can continue to show a different way of eating and moving with a goal set aside and distinct from that of changing the body. We can treat ourselves well simply because we deserve to be well.

I know that my body dysmorphic disorder will always be present, but I am now able to acknowledge it for what it is: untruths purported through my thoughts. I now understand that it is not an error with my body but rather an error of my mind. I know that these untrue thoughts will rise up in an effort to intimidate me at times, but I now have the tools to dissolve the thoughts that are not self-serving or self-loving. I know I will need to continue to be patient, continue to self-observe, and continue to plan for my personal well-being. I know each day will be different and some days will be hard. I know some days will not go as planned. But I also know all of this is okay. I have arrived in a place of self-acceptance and well-being. I am here, and now, I am free.

CHECKING IN

It is important to know that when you are practicing self-care your body becomes healthier internally. Picture your body healing from within each day as you incorporate these habits. Remind yourself that by living a healthier life you are creating a healthier body from within. Realize what it means to have a nourished body offering higher immunity from disease, less fatigue, more energy, better outlook, and generally feeling better in mind and body. Also, all bodies are intended to be different shapes and sizes and it is important to acknowledge, respect, and accept this fact. Realize that if you are truly caring for yourself there is so much more to benefit than some number on a scale. A great way to check in with yourself and set aside using body weight as the only check in is to answer the following questions:

- ❤ Are you truly working to deeply care for your body, mind, and soul?
- ❤ How is your body feeling; how is your mind feeling?
- ❤ What are your triggers/internal patterns causing actions that oppose self-care?
- ❤ Are there changes you want to make?
- ❤ What will you need to sustain self-care?

Checking in with your mind and body and listening to what they tell you will help guide you on the path of continued self-care.

STAYING ON THE PATH OF NOURISHMENT

The Sustainability Plan below will help you continue your self-care practice. You will find it familiar as it is a fresh version of your Wellness Plan. Set a specific time each week that you will check in with this plan. Make a point to release all-or-nothing thinking before it sets in. Commit to notice and release negative thought patterns when they set in as they are self-defeating. Rather, when life gets busy, I suggest utilizing your "If Nothing Else." Recall, this is something you know you can commit to when you aren't able to follow through with all your plans for self-care. An example may be "If Nothing Else, I will walk 15 minutes, meditate for 5 minutes, and eat vegetables or fruit with meals." Make sure your "If Nothing Else" is something that you know is very doable for you even when busy.

Sustainability Plan:

- ♥ What is your vision of wellness? (What would your world look like if you practiced self-caring actions?)
- ♥ What are your current barriers to your wellness vision? (What is currently preventing you from practicing self-care? What are your triggers or internal patterns that lead to behaviors opposing self-care?)
- ♥ What intention would you like to set? (Record a daily intention to help you stay present with this plan.)
- ♥ What behaviors/thoughts/habits will you change to help practice your intention? (Note: Dig deep and assess what need these behaviors are currently serving. Plan to meet this need in a way that better honors self-care and better serves you.)
- ♥ What changes will you make to your

environment to help practice your intention?

💜 What will help you make these changes? (Reflect on a typical day from wake to sleep and note what will help you.)

💜 What change beneficial to your physical, mental, or spiritual well-being will occur if you practice your intention?

💜 Now set a reminder to reflect weekly. Know that making adjustments/refinements in your plan as you continue to become self-aware is just fine. Keep this plan visible as a daily reminder. How will you recommit to your plan each day?

💜 How and where will you get support when you need it?

💜 What is your "If Nothing Else?"

If you recall in the beginning of this guide, we referred to some basic tenets to re-center you when you drift from your intention to care for yourself. They are noted again here:

💜 I have permission to live freely as my beautiful and authentic self.

💜 Happiness is always within me; I can support its manifestation through nourishment, movement, and connection to my inner wisdom.

- ♥ My value is constant, inherent, and infinite and not defined by anything externally sourced such as my appearance, comparison to others, or the opinion of others.
- ♥ I deserve to be well and my body deserves care as it is, in this moment.
- ♥ Rejuvenation starts with loving and caring action.

THANK YOU!

Thank you for allowing me to be with you along your self-care journey. I hope you have gained self-awareness and new knowledge that will continue to guide you with self-loving actions each and every day. And, above all, my hope is that now you are freely able to love yourself, treat yourself well, and finally … fully be well.

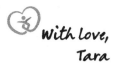

With love,
Tara

APPENDIX

BALANCED EATS

Vegetables & Fruit (½ Meal)		Grains & Starches (¼ Meal)	Protein (¼ Meal)	Healthy Fat (As a Side or Mixed in)
Vegetables	Fruits	Barley	Beans	Avocado/guacamole
Asparagus	Apples	Beans	Cheese	
Bell peppers	Applesauce	Bread	Edamame	Nuts
Broccoli	Bananas	Bulgar	Egg	Almonds
Brussel sprouts	Berries	Cereal	Fish	Cashews
Cabbage	Cantaloupe	Crackers	Kefir	Hazelnuts
Carrots	Cherries	Couscous	Lentils	Macadamia
Garlic	Dried fruit	Farro	Meat	Peanuts
Green beans	Figs	Kamut	Milk	Pecans
Jerusalem artichokes	Grapes	Millet	Nuts/nut butter	Pistachios
Leafy greens	Grapefruit	Oats	Poultry	Walnuts
Leeks	Kiwi	Pasta	Seeds/seed butter	
Mushrooms	Mango	Pita	Tempeh	Olives
Onions	Melon	Popcorn	Tofu	
Radishes	Orange	Rice	Yogurt	Oil
Scallions	Peaches	Quinoa		Avocado
Squash, summer	Pears	Tortilla		Olive
Sugar snap peas	Pineapples	Waffles		Peanut
Tomatoes	Plums	Wraps		etc.
Zucchini	Pomegranate			
		Starchy vegetables		Seeds
		Corn		Chia
		Peas		Flax
		Potatoes/sweet potatoes		Hemp
		Winter squash		Pumpkin
				Sunflower
				Sesame

EATING AWARENESS EXERCISE EXAMPLE

Day: Date:

Meal (generally describe what you ate, time of day and situation)	Hunger Level (type of hunger)	Emotions, sensations or thoughts prior to, during and after eating	Did emotions or situation feel tied to eating?	Did you choose your foods mindfully?	Did you practice embodied eating?	Did you enjoy this eating experience?
Example: Snack, Onion rings & milkshake; 3 PM. with kids in car	Extreme hunger	prior: anxious/stress, during: comforted, after: a little upset with myself	Yes, both situational and emotional hunger	I thought about it briefly before making the choice	No, I savored the taste, but I ate quickly and didn't pause to feel body	I did during but felt guilty and overfull after
Example: Breakfast, Overnight oats, almond butter; 8 AM, only one home	Initial to moderate hunger; feel that I made decision based on physical hunger	prior: relaxed, during: neutral, after: reflected on the eating experience	No	Yes. I planned the food the day prior and paused the day of before choosing	Yes, I connected to my inner wisdom throughout, took deep breaths, chewed food, etc	Yes, I tasted the food and felt satisfied

Continue to log meals throughout day and then at the end of the day record any notes or self-observations that you made.

SAMPLE GROCERY SHOPPING PLANNER

Dry goods section:

- ☐ _____
- ☐ _____
- ☐ _____
- ☐ Beans, variety dried or canned
- ☐ Bread, whole grain
- ☐ Crackers, whole grain
- ☐ Dark chocolate, 70% or higher cacao
- ☐ Dried fruit, no sugar added
- ☐ Grains, e.g. amaranth, barley, farro
- ☐ Herbs and spices, e.g. garlic, ginger, cayenne, cinnamon, turmeric
- ☐ Lentils
- ☐ Nut Butters, e.g. peanut, almond, or other, without hydrogenated oils
- ☐ Nuts, e.g. almonds, pistachios, walnuts
- ☐ Nutritional yeast
- ☐ Oats
- ☐ Oil, olive and avocado
- ☐ Pasta, whole grain
- ☐ Pepitas
- ☐ Popcorn
- ☐ Powder, e.g. cacao
- ☐ Quinoa
- ☐ Tea, green
- ☐ Tuna, water packed
- ☐ Seeds, e.g. chia, hemp, milled flax
- ☐ Sweetener, raw honey

Freezer section:

- ☐ _____
- ☐ _____
- ☐ _____
- ☐ Fish, wild caught salmon
- ☐ Fruit
- ☐ Meat, lean poultry
- ☐ Vegetables

Produce section:

- ☐ _____
- ☐ _____
- ☐ _____
- ☐ Fats, avocados
- ☐ Fruits examples:
    - ☐ Apples
    - ☐ Bananas
    - ☐ Berries, blackberries, blueberries, raspberries, strawberries
    - ☐ Cantaloupe
    - ☐ Cherries
    - ☐ Grapes
    - ☐ Grapefruit
- ☐ Kiwi
- ☐ Mangos
- ☐ Melon and watermelon
- ☐ Peaches
- ☐ Pineapples
- ☐ Plums
- ☐ Pomegranate
- ☐ Vegetables examples:
    - ☐ Asparagus
    - ☐ Bell peppers
    - ☐ Broccoli
    - ☐ Brussel sprouts
    - ☐ Cabbage, e.g. green or purple
    - ☐ Carrots
    - ☐ Garlic
    - ☐ Green beans
    - ☐ Jerusalem artichokes
    - ☐ Leafy greens, e.g. arugula, kale, microgreens, romaine, spinach
    - ☐ Leeks
    - ☐ Mushrooms, e.g. shiitake and vitamin D containing brands
    - ☐ Onions
    - ☐ Radishes
    - ☐ Scallions
    - ☐ Summer squash
    - ☐ Tomatoes
    - ☐ Zucchini
- ☐ Starchy vegetables:
    - ☐ Peas
    - ☐ Potatoes and sweet potatoes
    - ☐ Sweet corn
    - ☐ Winter squash

Refrigerator section:

- ☐
- ☐ _____
- ☐ _____
- ☐ Eggs, pasture raised
- ☐ Fermented food (especially those containing live cultures), kefir, kimchi, kombucha, miso, sauerkraut, tempeh, yogurt
- ☐ Fish, wild caught salmon
- ☐ Hummus
- ☐ Meat, lean poultry
- ☐ Milk, e.g. from grass fed cows or fortified plant milk
- ☐ Tofu

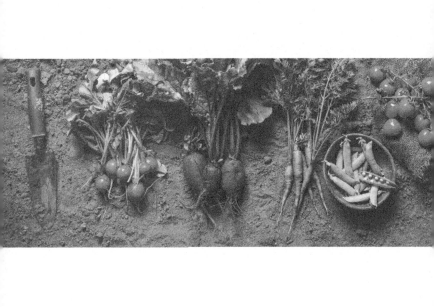

RECIPES

BREAKFAST RECIPES
Frittata Muffins
Yield: 12

Ingredients

- 1 tbsp avocado oil
- 2 tbsp garlic
- 1 cup asparagus, chopped
- ¼ cup green pepper, chopped
- 1/8 cup onion, chopped
- ¼ cup mushrooms, chopped
- ¼ cup olives of choice
- 6 eggs
- ½ cup milk
- ¼ tsp salt
- Ground black pepper to taste
- 1 cup shredded mozzarella

Instructions

- Preheat oven to 350 degrees F.
- In a skillet, heat avocado oil and garlic and add in the asparagus, green pepper, onion, mushrooms, and olives. Cook 5-10 minutes.

- ♥ Mix egg, milk, salt, and pepper in a mixing bowl and add vegetables from the skillet and the cheese.
- ♥ Spoon mixture into muffin tin approximately ¾ full per muffin.
- ♥ Bake about 20 minutes or until fully cooked through.

No-cook Oatmeal Smoothie

Ingredients (One serving—increase measurements for additional servings)

- ♥ ½ cup nut milk
- ♥ ½ cup old-fashioned rolled oats
- ♥ ½ cup yogurt (optional)
- ♥ 1 tsp chia seeds
- ♥ 1 tsp flaxseed milled
- ♥ 1 tsp hemp seeds
- ♥ ½ banana, mashed
- ♥ Fruit, nuts, and/or spices of preference to top
- ♥

Instructions

- ♥ Add milk, oats, yogurt, chia seeds, flaxseed, hemp seeds, and banana to a bowl and stir. Transfer to jar, place lid on jar and refrigerate for 5-8 hours.
- ♥ Remove from refrigerator, top with desired fruit, nuts, and/or spices and enjoy.

Whole Grain Lemon Blueberry Pancakes

Yield: 4-5

Ingredients

- 2 ripe bananas, mashed
- 2 eggs
- 1/2 cup whole-wheat flour
- 1/4 cup nut milk
- 1/2 tsp baking soda
- Small amount of avocado oil
- 1 cup fresh blueberries
- Zest and juice of 1 lemon
- Raw honey (optional)

Instructions

- In a bowl, mix evenly the bananas, eggs, flour, milk, lemon zest, lemon juice, and baking soda. Add some of the blueberries to the mix if you prefer.
- Coat a frying pan with oil and heat to medium. Add a small amount of pancake mix and cook until light brown. Then flip and cook to light brown on the other side. Do this until all the pancake mix is cooked.
- Top with the blueberries and honey if you would like.

Yogurt with Fruit and Seeds
Yield: 1

Ingredients (One serving—increase measurements for additional servings)

- ½ cup Greek vanilla yogurt
- 1 tbsp hemp seeds
- 1 tbsp chia seeds
- 1 tbsp flaxseed milled
- 1 tbsp cacao powder
- Berries (Raspberries pair nicely), nuts or nut butter, and/or spices of preference

Instructions

- Add yogurt, hemp seeds, chia seeds, flaxseed, and cacao powder to a bowl and stir.
- Fold in desired berries, nuts or nut butter, and/or spices and enjoy.

MEAL/SIDE RECIPES
Cherry & Pecan Farro
Yield: 6

Ingredients

- 1 1/2 cups farro
- 1/2 cup toasted chopped pecans
- 1/2 cup dried cherries
- 1/3 cup chopped scallions
- 1/4 cup chopped fresh parsley
- 2 tbsp lemon juice
- 2 tbsp olive oil

- ♥ 1/4 tsp salt
- ♥ 1/4 tsp black pepper
- ♥ 1/2 cup fresh mozzarella cubed

Instructions

- ♥ Boil approximately 4 cups water in a pot, add 1 1/2 cups uncooked farro.
- ♥ Cook the farro until tender, for about 15 minutes, stirring occasionally.
- ♥ Drain using a mesh colander, rinse under cold water, and place the well-drained farro in a medium bowl.
- ♥ Stir in the pecans, dried cherries, scallions, parsley, lemon juice, olive oil, salt, black pepper, and mozzarella cheese. Enjoy!

Coconut Curry Shrimp Noodle Bowl

Yield: 4-6

Ingredients

- ♥ 1-2 tbsp sesame oil
- ♥ 1 cup baby Bok choy, chopped
- ♥ 1 red pepper, diced
- ♥ ½ cup mushrooms, diced
- ♥ ½ cup shredded carrots
- ♥ 1 cup broccoli, chopped
- ♥ 1 cup edamame
- ♥ 4 cloves garlic, minced
- ♥ 1 tablespoon curry powder
- ♥ ¾ of 13 oz can unsweetened coconut milk

- ♥ 1 pound shrimp, cooked, peeled and deveined
- ♥ 2 cups cooked brown rice noodles
- ♥ Top with cilantro
- ♥ Serve with lime wedge

Instructions

- ♥ Heat the oil in a large skillet over medium-high heat. Add the shrimp and heat until warmed through.
- ♥ Add the garlic, vegetables, and curry powder to the skillet, cook for a few minutes to soften the vegetables, stirring periodically. Reduce the heat to medium-low, pour and stir in the coconut milk, and cook for several minutes until mixture is slightly thickened.
- ♥ Serve the shrimp and vegetables over the cooked rice noodles (be sure to get some of the liquid as well), squeeze the juice of a lime wedge over this, and top with cilantro.

Cranberry & Almond Quinoa

Yield: 6

Ingredients

- ♥ 1 1/2 cups quinoa
- ♥ 1/2 cup toasted sliced almonds
- ♥ 1/2 cup dried whole cranberries

- 1/3 cup chopped scallions
- 1/4 cup chopped fresh parsley
- 2 tbsp lemon juice
- 2 tbsp olive oil
- 1/4 tsp salt
- 1/4 tsp black pepper
- 1/2 cup feta cheese

Instructions

- Cook the quinoa according to package.
- Stir in the sliced almonds, dried cranberries, scallions, fresh parsley, fresh lemon juice, olive oil, salt and black pepper, and ½ cup feta cheese.
- Enjoy!

Fresh Avocado Salad

Yield: 6

Ingredients

- 2 ripe large avocados, diced
- 1 Vidalia onion, chopped
- 1 sweet bell pepper, chopped
- 1 tomato, chopped
- 1/3 cup fresh cilantro, chopped
- Juice from a lime

Instructions

- Combine all ingredients in a large bowl—mix and serve.

91

Garlic Herb Salmon

Yield: 4

Ingredients

- 4-5 garlic cloves, minced
- 1 tbsp minced fresh rosemary
- 2 tsp minced fresh thyme
- 4 tbsp avocado oil (plus a small amount to coat pan)
- Pinch of black pepper
- 4 salmon fillets (about 4 or so ounces each)
- 1 lemon

Instructions

- Heat oven to 375 degrees F.
- Lightly coat a baking pan with oil.
- In a small bowl, combine the minced garlic, herbs, pepper, and avocado oil, and mix well.
- Place the salmon fillets in the baking pan and coat them evenly with the garlic and herb mixture.
- Bake for approximately 20 minutes, until the fillets register 145 degrees F.
- Meanwhile, juice the lemon.
- Drizzle the baked salmon fillets with the lemon juice and enjoy.

Garlic-Parmesan Sweet Potato and Zucchini Noodles

Yield: 2

Ingredients

- ❤ 3 medium garlic cloves
- ❤ 3 tbsp avocado oil
- ❤ ¼ tsp crushed red pepper
- ❤ 1 medium zucchini
- ❤ 1 medium sweet potato
- ❤ 3 tablespoons grated parmesan cheese

Instructions

- ❤ Thinly slice the garlic.
- ❤ Cut off each end of the zucchini and sweet potato and then spiralize them (if you don't have a spiralizer you can pre-purchase veggie noodles). Trim the noodles with scissors and set aside.
- ❤ Place a large skillet on medium heat and pour in the oil. Add the garlic and crushed red pepper and cook for 30 seconds or until garlic is fragrant. Add in the sweet potato noodles and toss for approximately 5 minutes. Next add the zucchini noodles and toss for an additional 2-3 minutes or until preferred texture is achieved.
- ❤ Remove the skillet from the heat and toss in the parmesan cheese until melted. Serve immediately for best taste.

Half Moon Cabbage

Yield: 6

Ingredients

- 💜 1 head cabbage
- 💜 1-2 tbsp avocado oil
- 💜 Black pepper
- 💜 Garlic powder

Instructions

- 💜 Preheat oven to 425 degrees F.
- 💜 Remove loose leaves and hard base from the head of cabbage (to avoid waste: save loose cabbage for alternate use).
- 💜 Cut the head of cabbage in half and slice the cabbage into ½-inch-thick half-moons.
- 💜 Spread oil on the baking sheet.
- 💜 Place the half-moons on the baking sheet, brush the top of the cabbage with oil.
- 💜 Sprinkle the black pepper and garlic powder on the cabbage.
- 💜 Bake for 30 minutes or until the edges brown and become crispy. Serve immediately for best taste.

Immune Boost Chicken Soup Recipe

Yield: 8

Ingredients

- 💜 1 lb chicken breast, boneless, skinless
- 💜 15 oz can chickpeas, drained

- ❤ 3 cups broccoli, chopped
- ❤ 2 cups carrots, chopped
- ❤ 2 cups celery, chopped
- ❤ 1 cup kale, spines removed, chopped
- ❤ 1 red bell pepper, chopped
- ❤ 1 cup mushrooms, chopped
- ❤ 4 garlic cloves, minced
- ❤ 3 tbsp fresh ginger, chopped
- ❤ 1 medium onion, chopped
- ❤ 1/2 cup parsley
- ❤ 2 qt chicken broth
- ❤ 1/4 tsp crushed red pepper
- ❤ 1/2 tsp turmeric, ground
- ❤ 1 tsp curry powder
- ❤ 2 tbsp avocado oil
- ❤ Black pepper, dash

Instructions

- ❤ Add avocado oil, onion, celery, carrots, garlic, and ginger to a large pot and cook for 5 minutes to soften a bit.
- ❤ Add the chicken broth, raw chicken, turmeric, curry, crushed red pepper, and black pepper.
- ❤ Let boil. Then lower the heat to medium-low and simmer for about 20 minutes or until chicken breasts have cooked all the way through.
- ❤ Remove the chicken with tongs, shred

with 2 forks, then return to pot. Add the chickpeas, broccoli, red bell pepper, mushrooms, kale and parsley to the soup pot. Stir and simmer for an additional 15 minutes to soften the vegetables. Enjoy!

Lemon White Bean and Arugula Salad

Yield: 4

Ingredients

- ❤ 5 packed cups (5 ounces) arugula
- ❤ 1 (15-ounce) can cannellini beans, rinsed and drained
- ❤ 1/2 small red onion, thinly sliced
- ❤ 3 tbsp Kalamata olives, chopped
- ❤ 3 tbsp fresh lemon juice (about 1 large lemon)
- ❤ 1 tbsp raw honey
- ❤ 1 tsp lemon zest
- ❤ 3 tbsp extra-virgin olive oil
- ❤ Salt and freshly ground black pepper

Instructions

- ❤ In a large salad bowl, combine the arugula, beans, red onion, and olives.
- ❤ In a separate small bowl, mix the lemon juice, honey and lemon zest. Slowly whisk in the oil until combined. Season with salt and pepper.
- ❤ Pour the lemon mixture over the salad and mix to coat. Enjoy

Roasted Asparagus Recipe

Yield: 4

Ingredients

- 💜 12-15 small asparagus spears, rinsed and bottom ends trimmed
- 💜 1 tbsp garlic, minced (3 cloves)
- 💜 ¼ cup shaved parmesan cheese
- 💜 ¼ tsp pepper
- 💜 Avocado oil to coat

Instructions

- 💜 Preheat oven to 425 degrees F.
- 💜 Line a baking sheet with foil.
- 💜 Add the garlic, parmesan, and pepper together and set aside.
- 💜 Rub the asparagus to coat with oil and place spears close together on the baking sheet.
- 💜 Add the garlic-parm mixture to the asparagus, being careful to keep it on top the spears.
- 💜 Bake for 10 minutes and enjoy!

Sesame Kale

Yield: 4

Ingredients

- 💜 2 tsp sesame oil
- 💜 2 tsp reduced sodium tamari

- ❤ 4 packed cups kale, spines removed and broken into pieces
- ❤ Sesame seeds to coat

Instructions

- ❤ Massage the kale with the sesame oil and tamari.
- ❤ Sprinkle on sesame seeds, chill and enjoy!

Sesame-Maple Tempeh Lettuce Wraps

Yield: 6

Ingredients

- ❤ 3 tbsp sesame oil
- ❤ 16-ounces tempeh, crumbled
- ❤ 3 tbsp pure maple syrup
- ❤ 3 tbsp reduced-sodium soy sauce
- ❤ 2 tbsp water
- ❤ 1 ½ tbsp sesame seeds
- ❤ 1 ½ tbsp chia seeds
- ❤ 1 cup carrots, grated
- ❤ ½ cup dried cranberries
- ❤ 1 head of romaine lettuce

Instructions

- ❤ Combine maple syrup, soy sauce, water, chia seeds, and sesame seeds in a small mixing bowl. Let sit to thicken while completing next step.
- ❤ Heat the oil in skillet over medium-low

heat. Add tempeh and cook for approximately 10 minutes, stirring frequently.

♥ Reduce heat to low and add the maple syrup mixture to the skillet. Stir to coat the tempeh for about a minute.

♥ Add in the carrots and dried cranberries, stir and remove from heat.

♥ Place desired amount of tempeh mixture on a piece of romaine lettuce and enjoy.

Shitake Bean Patties

Yield: 8-10

Ingredients

♥ 2-3 tbsp avocado oil, split

♥ 1 yellow onion, chopped

♥ 4 garlic cloves, minced

♥ 1 cup shiitake mushrooms, stems removed, diced into small bits

♥ 1 tsp ground cumin

♥ 1 tbsp brown rice miso

♥ 1/4 tsp pepper

♥ 1 - 15 ounce can pinto beans, rinsed and drained

♥ 1 - 15 ounce can black beans, rinsed and drained

♥ 2 tbsp reduced sodium tamari

♥ 1-1/2 cups quick-cooking oats

♥ 8-10 whole grain hamburger buns

♥ 8 lettuce leaves

- ♥ 8 tomato slices
- ♥ Toppings of choice: mustard, ketchup, pickles, cheese

Optional—Miso Mayo

- ♥ 1 cup plain Greek yogurt
- ♥ ¼ cup brown rice miso
- ♥ 1 tbsp Dijon mustard

Instructions

- ♥ Heat the oil over medium heat in a skillet and sauté mushrooms, onion, and garlic for a couple minutes. Stir in the cumin and pepper and cook for 3 minutes. Remove the skillet from stove top.
- ♥ In a food processor, add pinto beans, black beans, miso, tamari, mushrooms/onion/garlic mixture, and oats. Pulse food processor to mix, ensuring to keep thick and chunky consistency.
- ♥ Shape mixture into patties. Add oil to skillet and fry patties over medium heat until browned, about 5-7 minutes on each side. (Note: If you don't want to prepare all patties at this time, freeze the additional for later).
- ♥ Serve on buns with lettuce, tomato, and additional toppings of choice. For optional miso mayo, combine all ingredients, stir, and spread on bun.

Strawberry Citrus Salad

Yield: 4

Ingredients

- 6 cups salad greens of choice
- 2 cups fresh strawberries, sliced
- 4 mandarin oranges, peeled
- ½ cup feta cheese
- ½ cup pistachios, shelled
- ½ cup dried blueberries
- Vinaigrette of choice to top (raspberry vinaigrette works well)

Instructions

- Evenly distribute greens onto 4 salad plates. Then evenly distribute the other ingredients on top.
- Add vinaigrette and enjoy!

Sweet Potatoes with Spicy Turmeric Tamari

Yield: 6

Ingredients

- 2 medium sweet potatoes cubed into ½ inch pieces
- 3 tbsp avocado oil
- 1 ½ tbsp honey
- 1 tbsp reduced-sodium tamari
- ½ tsp crushed chili peppers
- ½ tsp ground turmeric
- Pinch of pepper

- 3 tbsp dried sour cherries
- ¼ cup chopped pecans

Instructions

- Heat the avocado oil in a large skillet over medium-high heat. Add sweet potatoes, ensuring all sweet potatoes are touching the bottom of the skillet, cover, and cook approximately 4 minutes, stirring a couple of times. Uncover and reduce heat to medium-low and cook approximately 2-3 additional minutes.
- Meanwhile, combine honey, tamari, crushed chili pepper, turmeric, and pepper in a small bowl.
- Add the honey mixture, the pecans, and the cherries and simmer, stirring, for 30 seconds. Remove from heat.
- Transfer to bowl and enjoy warm.

Tandoori Tofu

Yield: 4

Ingredients

- 14 ounce block extra-firm tofu, drained and pressed to remove absorbed water
- 1-2 tbsp avocado oil (to stir fry in)
- 1 tbsp Tandoori spice blend
- 1 tbsp sesame seeds
- Handful or 2 of pea shoots
- Tamari or soy sauce to marinate

Instructions

- ♥ Cut the tofu into small bite-sized pieces, place in a bowl and marinate in tamari or soy sauce.
- ♥ Add oil to a pan and allow to heat for a couple minutes. Then add the tofu and sauté in the pan.
- ♥ While sautéing, add the pea shoots, tandoori, and sesame seeds.
- ♥ Cook until thoroughly heated, stirring occasionally.
- ♥ Serve warm!

SNACK RECIPES

Almond Rolled Chocolate Covered Strawberries

Yield: 12 Strawberries

Ingredients

- ♥ 12 large ripe strawberries, washed
- ♥ ¼ cup cacao powder
- ♥ ¼ cup coconut oil
- ♥ 2 tbsp honey
- ♥ ¼ tsp vanilla extract
- ♥ Almonds, chopped

Instructions

- ♥ Melt the coconut oil in saucepan then add the honey and vanilla.
- ♥ Slowly mix in the cacao powder until smooth.

- ♥ Transfer to bowl and allow to cool for a minute or so. Then dip the strawberries into the melted chocolate mixture and immediately roll in your chopped nuts.
- ♥ Keep in refrigerator until ready to serve.

Chocolate Cherry Black Bean Brownie Recipe

Yield: 16

Ingredients

- ♥ 1 ½ cups black beans
- ♥ 2 tbsp cacao powder
- ♥ 1/2 cup quick oats
- ♥ 1/4 cup honey
- ♥ 1/2 cup almond milk
- ♥ 2 tsp pure vanilla extract
- ♥ 1/2 tsp baking powder
- ♥ 1/3 cup chocolate chips (additional to top brownies)
- ♥ 1/3 cup dried cherries (additional to top brownies)

Instructions

- ♥ Preheat oven to 350 degrees F.
- ♥ In a food processor, blend all ingredients with the exception of the chocolate chips and dried cherries.
- ♥ Stir chocolate chips and dried cherries into the mixture.
- ♥ Pour mixture into a greased 8×8 pan.

Sprinkle extra chocolate chips and dried cherries over the top.

❤ Cook for 20 minutes, then let cool before trying to cut. Note: Brownies may appear gooey at first but will get a firmer once cool.

Crispy Kale
Yield: 2-3

Ingredients

❤ 4 cups kale, spines removed and broken into large pieces
❤ 2 tsp avocado oil
❤ 2 tsp tamari
❤ 3 tbsp nutrition yeast
❤ Salt (optional)

Instructions

❤ Preheat the oven to 400 degrees F.
❤ Massage the kale with the avocado oil and tamari. Then add nutritional yeast and a dash of salt if desired.
❤ Spread the kale in a single layer on a wax paper covered baking sheet.
❤ Make sure the oven has warmed for several minutes then place the baking sheet in the oven AND turn off the oven.
❤ Wait 20-25 minutes, then check for crispness. Remove the crispy pieced and leave

any damp pieces in the oven a bit longer before removing.

Turmeric Ginger Roasted Chickpeas

Yield: 4

Ingredients

- ♥ 15-ounce can chickpeas rinsed and drained
- ♥ ½ tbsp sesame oil
- ♥ ¼ tsp ground ginger
- ♥ ¼ tsp turmeric
- ♥ ¼ tsp garlic powder
- ♥ 1/8 tsp salt

Instructions

- ♥ Preheat oven to 400 degrees F.
- ♥ Rinse chickpeas and dry with paper towel.
- ♥ In a medium bowl, add oil, ginger, turmeric, garlic powder. Coat chickpeas in mixture.
- ♥ Bake the chickpeas on a baking sheet at 400 degrees F for 30minutes (stir at 15 minutes) or until brown and crispy. Use caution not to overcook or burn. Cool and enjoy.

Warm Peaches and Cream Recipe

Yield: 4

Ingredients

- ♥ 2 ripe peaches, halved, pitted, and cut into wedges

- ¼ cup balsamic vinegar
- ¾ cup pecans
- ¼ cup fresh mint leaves, chopped
- Avocado oil to coat pan
- 2 cups vanilla yogurt (frozen or regular), divided into 4 - ½ cup servings

Instructions

- Marinate the peach wedges in the balsamic vinegar.
- Add avocado oil to pan and cook the peaches, pecans, and mint on medium heat stirring periodically until warmed through and softened (approx. 7 minutes).
- While still warm, add the peaches and pecan mixture to top the yogurt.

More Snack Ideas

- Apple slices and nut butter
- Baked apples topped with cinnamon
- Banana ice cream—chop banana, freeze, puree (optional: add nut butter)
- Chocolate frozen yogurt sandwich - mix cocoa into yogurt, freeze in between whole grain graham crackers
- Cottage cheese and cantaloupe, mango, or other fruit
- Edamame
- Frozen banana—cut banana in half, coat

with plan Greek yogurt, put back together
with popsicle stick in the middle, freeze
- ♥ Grapes and cheese cubes
- ♥ Greek yogurt mixed with raw honey
- ♥ Jicama slices with salsa
- ♥ Kefir or yogurt berry smoothie
- ♥ Nuts and pomegranate mix
- ♥ Pepitas and dried cherries
- ♥ Popcorn cooked in avocado oil sprinkled with turmeric and nutritional yeast
- ♥ Small baked potato with salsa
- ♥ Tuna seasoned with pepper and turmeric on whole grain crackers or vegetable
- ♥ Whole grain cracker or vegetables and hummus
- ♥ Whole grain pita and cheese
- ♥ Yogurt mixed with chia seed and milled flax

ACKNOWLEDGEMENTS

Thank you to Sarah and Erin. *Love Body* would never have been what it is today without both of you. Thank you to Brooke L. Diaz, who thoughtfully edited this book. Thank you to my family for allowing me the time to practice what I preach.

ABOUT THE AUTHOR

Tara Rybicki received her Master of Science Degree in Nutrition from Central Michigan University. She has been a Registered Dietitian since 2003 and went on to gain further credentialing as a Certified Diabetes Educator. Her experience includes time in clinical inpatient and outpatient nutrition counseling, nutrition advisement, community health, as well as developing the Love Body Self-Care method. She is a mother of two girls, a wife to a Virgo, and a novice forager

Made in the USA
Monee, IL
23 February 2022

91715385R00077